Antibiotic/Antimicrobial Use in Dental Practice

Edited by

Michael G. Newman, D.D.S.

Adjunct Professor of Periodontics
School of Dentistry
University of California at Los Angeles Medical Center
Los Angeles, California

Kenneth S. Kornman, D.D.S., Ph.D.

Professor and Chairman
Department of Periodontics
Dental School
The University of Texas Health Sciences Center at San Antonio
San Antonio, Texas

Quintessence Publishing Co., Inc.
Chicago, Berlin, London, Tokyo, São Paulo, and Hong Kong

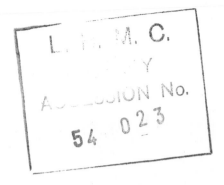
Library of Congress Cataloging-in-Publication Data

Antibiotic/antimicrobial use in dental practice / edited by Michael G.
  Newman, Kenneth S. Kornman.
      p.   cm.
    Rev. ed of: Guide to antibiotic use in dental practice. 1984.
    Includes bibliographical references.
    Includes index.
    ISBN 0-86715-172-2
    1. Antibiotics.   2. Materia medica, Dental.   I. Newman, Michael
G. II. Kornman, Kenneth S.   III. Guide to antibiotic use in dental
practice.
    [DNLM: 1. Antibiotics—adverse effects—handbooks.
2. Antibiotics—therapeutic use—handbooks.   3. Mouth Diseases—drug
therapy—handbooks.   4. Tooth Diseases—drug therapy—handbooks.
WU 39 G946]
RK715.A58G85   1990
617.6'061—dc20
DNLM/DLC   90-9099
for Library of Congress   CIP

quintessence
books

Books Editor: Laura G. Peppers
Production Manager: Kim Vander Steen
Production Editor: Kristen Trotter

Composition: Midwest Technical Publications, St. Louis, MO
Printing and binding: Edwards Brothers Inc, Ann Arbor, MI
Printed in USA

Dedication

We dedicate this book to our families. Their support and love have always been the encouragement we have sincerely appreciated and received.

PART 5: Special Considerations

Prophylactic Antibiotic Use *Otomo-Corgel/Sonis*

Antimicrobial Therapy for Immunocompromised Patients *Redding*

Systemic Considerations for Female Patients *Otomo-Corgel*

Legal Considerations *Zinman*

Contents

PART 1: GENERAL PRINCIPLES

CHAPTER 1

Orofacial Infections and Antibiotic Management 22

CHAPTER 2

Plaque-Associated Conditions 36

PART 2: DRUGS OF CHOICE

CHAPTER 3

Testing Antimicrobial Susceptibility 46

CHAPTER 4

Cultural Microbiology Sampling and Analysis   63

CHAPTER 5

Individual Drugs   68

CHAPTER 6

Topical Antimicrobial Agents: General Principles and Delivery Systems   89

CHAPTER 7

Topical Antimicrobial Agents: Individual Drugs   98

CHAPTER 8

Antifungal and Antiviral Agents   110

PART 3: ADVERSE REACTIONS

CHAPTER 9

Allergic and Other Sensitivity Reactions   116

CHAPTER 10

Adverse Microbiological Effects   129

PART 4: CLINICAL APPLICATION

CHAPTER 11

Antibiotics in Periodontal Therapy   136

CHAPTER 12

Antibiotics in Endodontic Therapy   148

CHAPTER 13

Antibiotics for Oral and Maxillofacial Infections   158

CHAPTER 14

Pediatric Considerations   172

CHAPTER 15

Chemotherapeutic Agents in Restorative Dentistry   178

CHAPTER 16

Antimicrobials in Implant Dentistry   187

PART 5: SPECIAL CONSIDERATIONS

CHAPTER 17

Prophylactic Antibiotic Use   202

CHAPTER 18

Antimicrobial Therapy for Immunocompromised Patients   211

CHAPTER 19

Systemic Considerations for Female Patients   217

CHAPTER 20

Legal Considerations   223

APPENDIXES

Contributors

J. Craig Baumgartner, D.D.S., Ph.D.
Chief of Microbiology, US Army Institute
    of Dental Research
Walter Reed Army Medical Center
Washington, D.C.

Sebastian G. Ciancio, D.D.S., F.I.C.D.
Chairman and Professor, Department of
    Periodontology
School of Dentistry
State University of New York
Buffalo, New York

James J. Crawford, M.A., Ph.D.
Professor of Oral Biology and Coordinator,
    Infection Control
Department of Endodontics
Director, Oral Microbiology Laboratory
School of Dentistry
University of North Carolina
Chapel Hill, North Carolina

Thomas F. Flemmig, Dr. med. dent.
Visiting Assistant Professor, Sections of
    Periodontics and Oral Biology
School of Dentistry
University of California at Los Angeles
Los Angeles, California

Perry Klokkevold, D.D.S.
Adjunct Assistant Professor, Section of
    Hospital Dentistry
School of Dentistry
University of California at Los Angeles
Los Angeles, California

Kenneth S. Kornman, D.D.S., Ph.D.
Professor and Chairman, Department of
    Periodontics
Dental School
The University of Texas Health Sciences
    Center
San Antonio, Texas

Robert Lindemann, D.D.S.
Assistant Professor, Special Patient Care
Section of Pediatric Dentistry
School of Dentistry
University of California at Los Angeles
    Medical Center
Los Angeles, California

Mahnaz Moussavi, D.D.S.
Microbiology Periodontal Research
    Laboratory
School of Dentistry
University of California at Los Angeles
    Medical Center
Los Angeles, California

Sushma Nachnani, M.S.
Research Associate
School of Dentistry
University of California at Los Angeles
    Medical Center
Los Angeles, California

Michael G. Newman, D.D.S.
Adjunct Professor of Periodontics
School of Dentistry
University of California at Los Angeles
    Medical Center
Los Angeles, California

Joan Otomo-Corgel, D.D.S., M.P.H.
Acting Head, Periodontal Residency
 Program
Veterans Administration Hospital
West Los Angeles, California
and
Adjunct Associate Professor, Section of
 Periodontics
School of Dentistry
University of California at Los Angeles
 Medical Center
Los Angeles, California

Larry J. Peterson, D.D.S., M.S.
Professor and Chairman, Oral and
 Maxillofacial Surgery
College of Dentistry
The Ohio State University
Columbus, Ohio

Spencer W. Redding, D.D.S., M.Ed.
Associate Dean for Advanced Education
 and Hospital Affairs
Dental School
The University of Texas Health Sciences
 Center
San Antonio, Texas

Mariano Sanz, M.D., D.D.S.
Professor and Chairman, Postgraduate
 Periodontics
School of Dentistry
Complutense University of Madrid
Madrid, Spain

Stephen T. Sonis, D.M.D., D.MSc.
Chief, Dental Service
Brigham and Women's Hospital
Boston, Massachusetts

John A. Sorensen, D.M.D., F.A.C.P.
Assistant Professor and Director of
 Postgraduate Prosthodontics
School of Dentistry
University of California at Los Angeles
Los Angeles, California

Edwin J. Zinman, D.D.S., J.D.
Periodontist and Attorney at Law
San Francisco, California

Introduction

The first edition of this book *(Guide to Antibiotic Use in Dental Practice)* emphasized the dramatic increase and interest in the use of antimicrobials in dental practice; this trend has continued. Antimicrobials and antibiotics are an integral part of dentistry. With more interest and use, more precise strategies and responsibilities have become integrated into the way we think and the way we practice.

This new edition, *Antibiotic/Antimicrobial Use in Dental Practice,* has refined and added new information and concepts that have emerged during the last 6 years. As before, we have assembled a group of internationally recognized experts to provide the most direct and pertinent information for application to clinical practice.

Chapters retained from the first edition have been updated, and several new areas have been added and emphasized.

A general principles chapter on *plaque-associated conditions* describes the infections and bacteriologically-associated complications that arise from plaque bacteria. These are among the most common situations we deal with in clinical practice. By describing the nature of plaque, a background is provided as a fundamental basis for using many of the systemic and topical agents available.

A completely new and expanded section on *topical agents* presents a comprehensive view of the bewildering array of agents in use today. The "what, why, and when to use" are discussed in a straightforward, practical approach, including information on a revolution in periodontal therapy involving devices for local controlled release of antimicrobials in the periodontal pocket.

The emergence of *implants* as an integral part of dentistry has provided an opportunity to incorporate antimicrobials into the maintenance and treatment of plaque-associated conditions as well as in peri-implant infections. An excellent approach and guide is provided to assist the practitioner.

The natural association and importance between restorative dentistry and periodontics is a primary discussion in a new chapter on *restorative dentistry considerations.* This chapter also provides up-to-date information and suggestions for infections occurring in patients who have removable prostheses.

The last 6 years have been witness to a dramatic increase in dental patients who have various systemic conditions. This new edition contains greatly expanded chapters on *premedication guidelines* and systemic disease complications requiring antibiotic and antimicrobial intervention. A new chapter on *immunocompromised patients,* including the management of AIDS patients and transplant patients, discusses the unique and important considerations associated with these patients.

This new edition also concludes, as before, with a useful and quick-access appendix section that consolidates information discussed in detail in other parts of the book. It is a valuable quick reference guide.

Acknowledgments

Our appreciation and thanks are extended to our excellent and supportive contributors. Their labor of love has made this book a truly unique and important adjunct to dental practice. This new edition was built on the foundations and vision of Dr. Anthony Goodman. We miss Dr. Goodman's challenge and guidance, but his spirit and goals are incorporated in every chapter.

Notice on drug information

The authors, editors, and publisher have endeavored to ensure the accuracy of the information, indications, and drug dosages in this book. However, readers are advised to consult product information inserts enclosed in drug packages.

PART 1

GENERAL PRINCIPLES

CHAPTER 1

Orofacial Infections and Antibiotic Management

James J. Crawford, Ph.D.

Infections of the orofacial tissues

How they begin   Most localized or progressive orofacial infections requiring antibiotic treatment occur when bacteria from dental plaque invade surrounding tissues. The
bacteria extend or displace through diseased teeth and supporting tissues, or after
accidental or clinical trauma. Cariogenic microorganisms can spread through dentin
and infect the pulp space and periapical tissues. Facultative and anaerobic plaque
bacteria proliferate in the gingival and periodontal tissues to cause several types of
infections, including periodontitis, ulcerative gingivitis, and pericoronitis. Bacteria
carried from the gingival sulci and pockets by the blood can infect nonvital pulps in
noncarious, intact teeth and can cause bacteremia and septicemia. Compound fractures,
periodontal surgery, exodontia, and other types of tissue trauma can also introduce
enough plaque bacteria into tissues to cause severe infections.[1-7]

The body's response   Acute inflammation caused by invading bacteria will cause
polymorphonuclear leukocytes to accumulate in the infected area, forming an exudate
that may be detectable as pus. The infection is then called **purulent.** The infective
microorganisms are called pyogenic—pus-producing—even though the purulence is
primarily a host response, triggered by release of chemotactic substances and antigens
from the microorganisms.
   Often when the area of pus is walled off by fibrin deposition, an **abscess** develops.
Sometimes a more diffuse inflammation, called **cellulitis,** occurs. The two states are
not mutually exclusive. Many small foci of pus can exist in cellulitis, and the area
around a well-defined abscess is likely to be inflamed with more extravascular fluid than
is normal. Whether an inflammation is predominantly abscessed or cellulitic helps
determine diagnosis and treatment.

Types of infection

Infections can occur in soft tissue, in bone, and on exposed surfaces.

Internal infections

In purulent soft- or hard-tissue infections the exudate tends to migrate to the nearest area of least resistance, where it may erupt and drain. A chronic draining sinus tract may also develop. Less frequently, exudates that accumulate rapidly extend along fascial planes to involve other vital tissues or organs, providing a more immediate threat to the life of the host.[1] Antibiotics are usually required in both cases.

Mandibular infections   Progressive mandibular infections can produce:

1. Sublingual infections (Ludwig's angina) that involve submental spaces and cause edema of the pharynx and strangulation
2. Extension down into the mediastinum, where massive infection of the lungs or pericarditis can result

Maxillary infections   Extension of maxillary infections can result in critical conditions:

1. Cellulitis or abscesses can form in the orbits.
2. The cavernous sinus of the brain can become infected. The common oral pathogens, the black-pigmented *Bacteroides (Porphyromonas)** sp., including *Bacteroides gingivalis, Bacteroides intermedius, Bacteroides melaninogenicus,* and *Bacteroides endodontalis,* can lead to brain infection when the heparinase they produce causes thrombi to form. The thrombi can occlude facial veins, causing blood to flow back through valveless veins to the cranium and over the brain by way of emissary veins. Infected thrombi that dislodge and enter the circulation can lodge on the brain and cause abscesses to form on it. Resulting brain damage can be recognized by neurological symptoms. Infected thrombi can similarly become lodged in the cavernous sinus and, if massive enough, can cause death despite rigorous therapy.
3. The maxillary sinus can become infected.

*Editor's note: all oral black-pigmented *Bacteroides* are in the process of being reclassified and will no longer be called *Bacteroides* but will retain the current species name. For example, *Bacteroides gingivalis* will be renamed *Porphyromonas gingivalis.* In this edition reclassification is in a transition phase and the name *Bacteroides* has been retained.

Superficial infections

Superficial mucosal infections include:

1. Infections of exposed bone
2. Fungal stomatitis (candidiasis, thrush), caused by *Candida albicans* for which specific antifungal therapy is available (see chapters 5 and 8)
3. Acute necrotizing ulcerative gingivitis or gingivostomatitis, for which antibiotic therapy may or may not be part of treatment (see chapters 2 and 11)
4. Primary and tertiary syphilis, management of which should be referred to a physician trained in infectious diseases
5. Primary herpetic gingivostomatitis, in which prophylactic antibiotic administration (usually penicillin) may be considered to prevent secondary bacterial infection (acyclovir, an antiviral agent, is useful in relieving symptoms of primary herpes infections but is of limited efficacy in preventing recurrences; see chapter 8)
6. Recurrent herpetic lesions, which, because they are viral, do not respond to the antibiotics presently available
7. Aphthous ulcers and angular chelitis, which, while they may be primarily or secondarily infected with bacteria, are generally considered too trivial for systemic antibiotic treatment (Angular chelitis can be caused by *C. albicans* or *Staphylococcus aureus* and can remain chronic in older denture patients. Topical antibiotic ointments are usually effective for treating *S. aureus* infections; nystatin ointment is effective for treating *C. albicans* infections)

Types of bacteria in pyogenic orofacial infections

Anaerobic mixtures   Most bacteria in odontogenic or oral infections belong to anaerobic species similar to those found in plaque. They occur most often in mixtures of from two to six species (see **Tables 1.1 to 1.3**).

Some older texts wrongly attribute most oral infections exclusively to facultative pathogens such as *S. aureus,* coliform bacteria, and even *Streptococcus pyogenes* (the agent of bacterial pharyngitis, scarlet fever, and rheumatic fever). Such reports were probably due to contaminated samples and/or inappropriate culture technology, combined with a lack of comprehensive studies. Today we know that a mixture of facultative indigenous oral streptococci and anaerobic species, especially the *Bacteroides, Fusobacterium,* anaerobic cocci, and *Actinomyces* sp., are the most common agents of pyogenic submucosal orofacial infections. It has not been determined whether the detection by researchers of slow-growing *Actinomyces* in progressive, rapidly acute pyogenic infections is significant.

In 1980 Kannangara and associates studied the flora of 61 hospitalized patients with pyogenic infections of dental origin that were refractile to treatment.[8] *Bacteroides fragilis* was detected in nearly 30% of samples identified by the hospital laboratory.

Table 1.1 Bacteria in odontogenic and oral infections*

	Infection type				Root canals of necrotic teeth with lesions	
Organism	Perimandibular space infections⁴	Periapical abscesses in children⁹	Orofacial odontogenic infections¹	Bacteremia from tooth extraction¹⁰	Goodman study⁶	Sundqvist study⁷
Aerobic (facultative)						
Eikenella corrodens	+	–	–	–	–	–
Staphylococcus	+	–	–	–	–	–
Streptococcus	+	+	+	+	+	+
Anaerobic (obligate)						
Actinomyces	+	+	+	+	+	+
Bacteroides						
fragilis	–	–	++	++	+	–
melaninogenicus†	+	++	++	++	++	++
oralis	+	+	++	+	+	++
Bifidobacterium	–	–	++	–	+	++
Eubacterium	+	++	++	–	+	++
Fusobacterium	+	++	++	++	+	++
Peptococcus	+	++	++	++	+	++
Peptostreptococcus	+	+	++	+	+	+
Propionibacterium	+	–	+	+	+	+
Veillonella	+	+	+	+	+	+

*Partial listing of representative bacteria commonly encountered.
†Isolates listed in the original references and above as *B. melaninogenicus* most likely include *Bacteroides gingivalis*, *Bacteroides intermedius*, *B. melaninogenicus*, and *Bacteroides endodontalis*.

Table 1.2   Frequency of bacteria in oral infections

Organism	Bacteria secondary to tooth extraction[10]	Perimandibular space infections[4]	Periapical abscesses in children[9]	Orofacial odontogenic infections[1]	Root canals of necrotic teeth with lesions	
					Goodman study[6]	Sundqvist study[7]
			%			
Aerobic (facultative)						
Eikenella corrodens	0	15	0	0	0	0
Streptococcus	47	33	10	21	23	16
Staphylococcus	0	14	0	0	0	0
Anaerobic (obligate)						
Actinomyces	20	19	5	0	4	27
Bacteroides						
fragilis	4	0	0	10	7	0
melaninogenicus*	56	42	15	42	5	39
oralis	20	19	5	7	21	22
Bifidobacterium	0	0	0	0	2	0
Eubacterium	0	38	2	14	2	38
Fusobacterium	44	33	8	28	5	50
Peptococcus	16	52	20	0	9	38
Peptostreptococcus	24	0	7	57	18	27
Propionibacterium	12	19	0	0	22	16
Veillonella	20	14	75	7	34	11

*Isolates listed in the original references and above as *B. melaninogenicus* most likely include *Bacteroides gingivalis*, *Bacteroides intermedius*, *B. melaninogenicus*, and *Bacteroides endodontalis*.

Table 1.3 Organisms in acute orofacial infections*
Predominant organisms (detected in 126 samples)

Lesion category†	Anaerobic organisms‡	Aerobic facultative and capnophilic organisms
Abscess (46/126) 37%	Bacteroides melaninogenicus (16/46) 16% B. melaninogenicus ss. melaninogenicus (3/46) 7% B. melaninogenicus ss. intermedius (1/46) 2% Bacteroides asaccharolyticus (2/46) 4% Bacteroides uniformis (1/46) 2% Bacteroides sp. (19/46) 42% Fusobacterium nucleatum (2/46) 4% Fusobacterium sp. (1/46) 2% Veillonella parvula (3/46) 7% Peptostreptococcus parvula (1/46) 2% Peptostreptococcus anaerobius (1/46) 2% Peptostreptococcus micros (1/46) 2% Peptostreptococcus sp. (1/46) 2% Propionibacterium acnes (1/46) 2% Anaerobic gram positive rods (2/46) 4%	Streptococcus intermedius (2/46) 4% Streptococcus mitis (1/46) 2% Streptococcus viridans (26/46) 57% Streptococcus fecalis (1/46) 2% Streptococcus, group B (1/46) 2% Staphylococcus aureus (1/46) 2% Klebsiella pneumoniae (3/46) 7%
Post-surgical and extraction wounds (32/126) 25%	B. melaninogenicus ss. melaninogenicus (3/32) 9% B. melaninogenicus ss. intermedius (1/32) 3% B. asaccharolyticus (1/32) 3% Bacteroides sp. (6/32) 19% V. parvula (1/32) 3% Actinomyces viscosus (1/32) 3%	S. mitis (2/32) 6% Streptococcus sanguis (1/32) 3% S. viridans (10/32) 31% Streptococcus, group B (1/32) 3% S. aureus (3/32) 9% S. intermedius (3/32) 9% Eikenella corrodens (3/32) 9% Pseudomonas aeruginosa (2/32) 6% Enterobacter cloacae (1/32) 3% Enterobacter aerogenes (2/32) 6% Escherichia coli (2/32) 6% Klebsiella oxytoca (1/32) 3% K. pneumoniae (1/32) 3% Klebsiella sp. (1/32) 3%

*Other organisms often occur. See chapters 12 and 13 of this handbook for additional discussion of representative flora in specific infection types. Species names have been retained from the original reference.
†(Number of lesions out of total specimens) and percentage.
‡(Number of specimens from which isolated in each lesion category) and percentage.

Table 1.3 continues

Table 1.3   continued

Lesion category†	Anaerobic organisms‡	Aerobic facultative and capnophilic organisms
Endodontically involved infections (25/126) 20%	B. melaninogenicus (1/25) 4% B. melaninogenicus ss. intermedius (1/25) 4% B. uniformis (1/25) 4% Bacteroides capillosus (1/25) 4% Bacteroides sp. (4/25) 16% F. nucleatum (1/25) 4% V. parvula (1/25) 4% Peptococcus saccharolyticus (1/25) 4% Actinomyces odontolyticus (1/25) 4% Actinomyces sp. (1/25) 4% Anaerobic gram positive rods (2/25) 8%	S. sanguis (1/25) 4% S. viridans (12/25) 48% S. fecalis (2/25) 8% S. intermedius (1/25) 4% K. pneumoniae (1/25) 4%
Sinus tracts (16/126) 13%	B. melaninogenicus (2/16) 13% B. asaccharolyticus (1/16) 6% B. capillosus (1/16) 6% Bacteroides sp. (1/16) 6% Capnocytophaga sp. (1/16) 6% P. saccharolyticus (1/16) 6% P. anaerobius (1/16) 6% Actinomyces sp. (2/16) 13% V. parvula (1/16) 6%	S. intermedius (1/16) 6% S. viridans (6/16) 38% E. corrodens (1/16) 6% P. aeruginosa (1/16) 6% K. pneumoniae (2/16) 13%
Cellulitis (10/126) 8%	B. melaninogenicus (2/10) 20% B. asaccharolyticus (1/10) 10% Bacteroides sp. (3/10) 30% F. nucleatum (1/10) 10% Peptostreptococcus sp. (1/10) 10% Anaerobic gram positive rods (1/10) 10%	S. viridans (8/10) 80%
Surface lesion (6/126) 5%		Candida albicans (3/6) 50% normal flora only: Streptococcus and Neisseria sp. (3/6) 50%
Traumatic injuries (6/126) 5%	B. melaninogenicus (2/6) 33% Bacteroides sp. (1/6) 17% Actinomyces sp. (1/6) 17%	S. mitis (1/6) 17% S. viridans (1/6) 17% Capnocytophaga sp. (1/6) 17% K. oxytoca (1/6) 17%
Osteomyelitis (5/126) 4%	B. melaninogenicus ss. intermedius (1/5) 20% B. asaccharolyticus (1/5) 20% Bacteroides ureolyticus (1/5) 20% Bacteroides sp. (1/5) 20% P. saccharolyticus (1/5) 20% Actinomyces sp. (1/5) 20%	S. viridans (2/5) 40% Capnocytophaga sp. (1/5) 20%

Table 1.3 continued

Lesion category†	Anaerobic organisms‡	Aerobic facultative and capnophilic organisms
Cyst related infections (3/126) 2%		S. mitis (1/3) 33% S. viridans (2/3) 67%
Periodontally involved infections (2/126) 2%	Bacteroides sp. (2/2) 100%	
Human bite (1/126) 0.8%		S. mitis (1/1) 100% S. sanguis (1/1) 100%

Details of the extent of classification were not given. That the patients were all hospitalized with refractile infections suggests this was a group selected by those circumstances; it does not make them typical of the broad numbers of general outpatient surgery, endodontic, or periodontal practice patients who develop infections. However, the findings do reflect the problems encountered with refractile infections among hospitalized patients and deserve careful consideration.

Infection management

Drainage and debridement The essential features of infection management are drainage and debridement of the affected tissues. **Unless the source of the infection is removed, other modes of therapy will ultimately fail.**[1-3] Drainage is essential in therapy for pus-producing infections. It should be the first step in treatment.

The function of antibiotics Antibiotics may not always be bacteriocidal in the doses administered in dental practice. They are usually bacteriostatic, inhibiting bacterial metabolism and multiplication. In severely ill patients antibiotics can be administered in large enough doses to achieve bacteriocidal levels, usually by intravenous infusion. Such use requires careful supervision. In the mixed-bacterial infections most commonly found in the oral cavity, success of treatment does not depend on antibiotic effectiveness against *all* microorganisms present. The body can usually eliminate infection when an antibiotic inhibits metabolism and multiplication of the *predominant* pathogenic microorganisms.

Patient monitoring   Antibiotics usually only suppress an infection while the body begins to heal itself. Fluid, nutrition, rest, and adequate control of symptoms are necessary for this healing to begin and to continue.

Antibiotics cannot work miracles. They cannot prevent further debilitation of a patient who is rapidly deteriorating as fever and lack of food affect the health of the rest of the body. Hospitalization, intravenous supportive care, or general or specialized medical consultation may be required in cases of severe infection and debilitation. To determine this the patient's condition should be carefully monitored with respect to severity of the infection, rate of recovery, dehydration, debilitation, and contributing systemic factors.

Detailed clinical concepts of managing periapical infections have been well addressed elsewhere.[11,12] See also chapters 12 and 13.

The decision to use antibiotic therapy

Accounting for the risks

Antibiotics are often beneficial and even lifesaving in medical and dental therapy. *The decision to use antibiotics should be based on a thorough history, physical examination, laboratory data, and a diagnosis. Record all information in the chart, for effective patient management and legal purposes* (see chapter 20). *Also list the treatment provided, drugs prescribed, and directions given to the patient. Antibiotic therapy should also be supported by appropriate, prior, or supplementary laboratory culture evaluation.*[13]

The decision to use antibiotics should be carefully weighed with regard to the ratio of risks versus benefits. Antibiotics can cause severe allergic reactions or have toxic side effects. Their adverse effects include selection of resistant strains, resulting in adverse overgrowth of infectious yeasts or bacteria. Notable is intestinal overgrowth of *Clostridium dificile* resulting in pseudomembraneous cholitis. (Adverse reactions are covered in chapter 10.) However, not using an appropriate antibiotic when indicated to control an infection in the head and neck area can have serious consequences. Generalists should refer patients with severe infections to well-qualified specialists or to a hospital dentistry clinic where full laboratory and supportive care are available.[14]

Indications for prescribing antibiotics

It is most important that an antibiotic be used to treat an infection *(1)* if it seems likely that withholding the antibiotic will result in failure to effectively manage a severe or potentially life threatening infection, and *(2)* when the patient is immunocompromised or is at increased risk because of a systemic condition. Use of antibiotics should be based on clinical evaluation and the judgement that antimicrobial therapy will have a beneficial or therapeutic effect. Therapy should help contain and limit further extension of the infection, shorten duration of the infection and discomfort, or reduce risks of systemic involvement or complications.

Antibiotics should definitely be considered for patients with orofacial infections when one or more of the following related signs, symptoms, or conditions are present:

1. Fever and or chills, current or in the last 24 hours
2. Malaise, fatigue, weakness, dizziness, rapid respirations, or other debilitation
3. Trismus
4. Cellulitis; infection extending acutely (e.g., within the last 24 hours) into adjacent spaces or tissues without clearcut localization
5. Local or systemic infection with history of rheumatic fever, endocarditis, heart prosthesis, or other predisposing factors (chapter 17 details prophylactic antibiotic use)
6. Immunocompromised status (e.g., AIDS, cancer, autoimmune disease, corticosteroid therapy); see chapter 18
7. Allograph (cardiac, renal, bone marrow, liver and/or osseous implant)
8. Diabetes mellitis type I, II, or III or other contributory systemic disease

When an antibiotic is indicated the goal is to choose a drug that is selectively active against the most likely infecting agents and that has the least potential to cause allergic or toxic reactions in the specific patient under treatment.

Situations in which antibiotic therapy is not necessary

In persons *without abnormal systemic risks,* clinical experience has shown that antibiotics are not necessary for certain conditions and infections, such as:

1. Uncomplicated edema induced by trauma or chemicals (e.g., endodontic irrigating solutions)
2. Pain related to pulpitis or trauma
3. Well localized minor abscess that is likely to respond well to drainage and treatment of the local source of the infection, such as a periapical abscess
4. Chronic uncomplicated draining sinus tract associated with a nonvital tooth
5. Bacteria limited to a root canal
6. Uncomplicated dry socket
7. Simple, well-confined pericoronitis

Culture taking and susceptibility testing

When the decision is made to use an antibiotic as part of therapy for **serious infection**, the dentist should take a bacterial culture and submit it for identification and susceptibility testing. Chapters 3 and 4 cover collection technique and interpretation of results.

A **culture** detects and identifies the organisms that predominate in the sample when it arrives at the testing laboratory. **Susceptibility testing** provides in vitro information on the susceptibility of organisms to particular antibiotics.

Therapy should not be delayed   In an acute, potentially serious situation, the need for immediate antibiotic therapy in conjunction with debridement rules out waiting for test results. The reasonable course of action is to take a bacteriological sample and at the same time to begin therapy with the antibiotic most likely to succeed (usually a penicillin; see chapter 5). If this therapy has not succeeded within 2 to 4 days, concrete bacteriological information from the laboratory will be available from the initial culture and susceptibility testing. Alternative therapy decisions can be based on this information. Delaying sampling until the infection fails to respond wastes time and money and places the patient at much greater risk.

If an infection is naturally draining in the absence of antibiotics but is not progressing toward healing, the dentist should take a bacterial specimen for laboratory analysis and at the same time prescribe penicillin (for penicillin-allergic patients, see chapter 5). Culture results will enable the dentist to alter the drug and provide the dosage best suited for the situation. Meanwhile, the most universally accepted drug for combating infection will have been provided in the interim.

Cost cannot be a factor in the decision to seek laboratory information; if antibiotic therapy and management are considered necessary, then so is the expense of appropriate testing, care, and laboratory followup.

Choosing the antibiotic therapy

Drug   Of the hundreds of antibiotics marketed and the 20 or so true generic forms available, only a limited number of antibiotics are needed in dental practice. Their properties and spectra are discussed in detail in chapter 5.

Dosage   **The only true guide to dosage is the response of the patient.** General dosage guidelines are found in chapter 5. Dosage varies directly with body weight and is modified by medical status and severity of the infection. As a general principle, it is wiser to chance prescribing too high a dosage. Too low a dose may cause treatment to fail, while too high a dose carries only a slightly greater risk of toxicity, and no greater risk of allergy induction.

Duration   Clinical remission is the primary guide to how long therapy should last. **Treatment should continue for at least 3 days after major symptoms subside**, to prevent rebound infection. This means that 5 days of therapy is the usual minimum, since the patient should show some improvement of a moderate infection after 1 or 2 days of therapy. Under severe conditions the patient might show only reduced fever and/or feel only somewhat better within this time. Extensive cellulitis, abscessed tissues, or infected bone can require 7 or more days of the therapy. It is imperative to treat the source of these infections and to establish drainage if appropriate. Osteomyelitis may require several weeks of specific antibiotic therapy in conjunction with other treatment modalities such as hyperbaric oxygen therapy (see chapter 13).

If response and recovery are slow, all aspects of treatment and diagnosis, as well as the patient's systemic health and defenses, should be reexamined. Patients must be strongly advised to continue therapy until the prescribed course is complete; it is the dentist's responsibility to monitor clinical progress (see chapter 20).

Why antibiotic therapy may fail

1. The patient does not comply with the prescription.
2. The dose prescribed is insufficient, or it is prescribed or taken for an insufficient duration.
3. An inappropriate antibiotic is prescribed.
4. The antibiotic is taken simultaneously with an interfering drug (e.g., an antacid with a tetracycline).
5. Drainage is inadequate or necrotic tissues have not been located and removed.
6. The predominant causative bacteria are resistant, resistant strains emerge, or the tissues become secondarily infected with resistant bacteria.
7. The antibiotic fails to reach the infected site (osteomyelitis).
8. A duct, such as a salivary gland, is obstructed or there is an open portal, such as for a urinary catheter or intravenous line.
9. Poor host response, such as malabsorption, is encountered due to a systemic disease.
10. The patient is reacting to a foreign body, such as a transplanted organ or an implant.

Common errors in antibiotic therapy

1. Viral infections cannot be treated with antibiotics.
2. Ineffective levels of the appropriate drug are administered.
3. A drug that has no established specific effectiveness is prescribed.
4. The infecting agent is not documented.
5. Toxic agents are used when less toxic medication would suffice.
6. Expensive drugs are prescribed when effective inexpensive drugs would suffice.
7. Antibiotic therapy is changed too rapidly and incorrectly, assuming therapeutic failure prior to correcting all contributing factors.
8. Cultures are not taken and susceptibility tests are not obtained.
9. The patient's progress is not monitored.

Points to remember

1. Antibiotics should not be used unless the need for them is certain.
2. An adequate health history, especially pertaining to allergies and toxic effects, must be taken prior to therapy.
3. Less than the recommended therapeutic dose should never be prescribed.

4. Administration one-half hour before meals or 2 to 3 hours after meals is advisable for optimal uptake of most antibiotics. Some antibiotics should be taken with meals, to avoid nausea.
5. There should be a prompt response that is beneficial, usually within 24 to 48 hours.
6. Therapy should be continued 3 days past the asymptomatic point.
7. If an antibiotic fails, do not hesitate to use other antibiotic therapy or dosage, *based on susceptibility testing*. This requires culturing exudates, where possible, before initiating therapy with the first agent.
8. Attention must be paid at all times to the possible development of adverse effects.

References

1. Chow, A.W., Roser, S.M., and Brady, F.A. 1978. Orofacial odontogenic infections. *Ann. Intern. Med.* 88:392–402.

2. Crawford, J.J. 1982. Periapical infections and infections of oral facial tissues. pp. 786–814. *In* J.R. McGhee et al. (eds.) *Dental Microbiology.* New York: Harper & Row.

3. Bartlett, J.G., and Gorbach, S. 1976. Anaerobic infections of the head and neck. *Otolaryngol Clin. North Am.* 9:655.

4. Bartlett, J.G., and O'Keefe, P. 1979. The bacteriology of perimandibular space infections. *J. Oral Surg.* 37:407–409.

5. Brook, I., and Finegold, S.M. 1978. Acute suppurative parotitis caused by anaerobic bacteria: Report of 2 cases. *Pediatrics* 62:1019–1020.

6. Goodman, A.D. 1977. Isolation of anaerobic bacteria from the root canal systems of necrotic teeth by the use of a transport solution. *Oral Surg.* 43:766–770.

7. Sundqvist, G.K. 1976. Bacteriologic studies of necrotic dental pulps. Odontological Dissertation No. 7, University of Umea, Umea, Sweden.

8. Kannangara, D.W., Thadepalli, H., and McQuirtir, J.L. 1980. Bacteriology and treatment of dental infections. *Oral Surg.* 50:103–109.

9. Brook, I., Grimm, S., and Kielich, R.B. 1981. Bacteriology of acute periapical abscess in children. *J. Endodontol.* 7:378–380.

10. Crawford, J.J. 1974. Bacteremia after tooth extraction studied with the aid of prereduced anaerobically sterilized culture media. *Appl. Microbiol.* 27:927–932.

11. Hooley, J.R., and Whitacre, R.J. (eds.) 1983. *Diagnosis and Treatment of Odontogenic Infections.* Seattle: Stoma Press.

12. Peterson, L.J., et al. (eds.) 1988. *Contemporary Oral and Maxillofacial Surgery.* St. Louis: The C.V. Mosby Co.

13. Hill, M.K., and Sanders, C.V. 1988. Principles of antimicrobial therapy for head and neck infections. *Infect. Dis. Clin. North Am.* 2:57–83.

14. Blomquist, I.K., and Bayer, A.S. 1988. Life threatening deep facial space infections of the head and neck. *Infect. Dis. Clin. North Am.* 2:237–264.

Further reading

AMA Drug Evaluations. 1977. 3rd ed. Littleton, Mass.: Publishing Sciences Group, Inc.

Kaye, D. 1983. Bacterial diseases. pp. 155–121. *In* L.F. Rose and D. Kaye (eds.) *Internal Medicine for Dentistry.* 1st ed. St. Louis: The C.V. Mosby Co.

Mandell, G.L., Douglas, R.G., and Bennett, J.E. 1979. *Principles and Practice of Infectious Diseases.* New York: John Wiley & Sons.

Medical Letter on Drugs and Therapeutics, 56 Harrison St., New Rochelle, N.Y.

Sande, M.A., and Mandell, G.L. 1980. Antimicrobial agents: general considerations. pp. 1080–1105. *In* A.G. Gilman et al. (eds.) Goodman and Gilman's *The Pharmacological Basis of Therapeutics.* 6th ed. New York: Macmillan Publishing Co.

CHAPTER 2

✓ Plaque-Associated Conditions

Mariano Sanz, M.D., D.D.S.

Caries and periodontal disease are the most prevalent infections in humans. These infections are caused by specific members of a large population of microorganisms in the oral cavity that form dental plaque. The term **dental plaque** is used universally to describe the association of bacteria to the tooth surface (see **Table 2.1**).

The oral cavity is a unique host environment that possesses ecological features that facilitate the establishment and growth of a great variety of microorganisms including bacteria, fungi, viruses, and protozoa. These ecologic mechanisms permit the colonization of oral bacteria in a predictable succession. If this microbial community on tooth surfaces is prevented from maturing, it may be compatible with gingival and dental health. However, if it is allowed to grow and mature it usually produces inflammatory changes in the periodontal tissues. Imbalances in host defenses or disturbances in the oral ecological environment will facilitate opportunistic infections by indigenous and exogenous microorganisms. These may be life threatening in special patients or

Table 2.1 Plaque-associated conditions

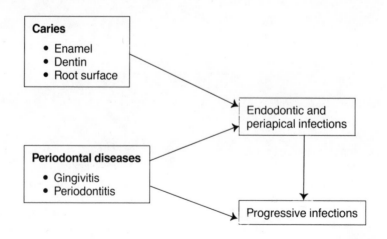

situations. In order to treat these microbe-related conditions, it is important to have a thorough understanding of the specific factors involved in their etiology and course.

Oral microflora

The oral environment has unique ecological characteristics such as temperature, humidity, and a wide variety of constantly supplied nutrients that allow the colonization and growth of many nutrients, which in turn allow the colonization and growth of a great number of microorganisms. There may be over 200 different species that can be isolated from dental plaque alone. From this, the *indigenous flora* comprise those species that are almost always present in high numbers and are compatible with the host and therefore do not compromise host survival. Within the oral cavity, different environmental conditions will selectively contribute to the specific microflora. The microbial population that forms on the surfaces of teeth (plaque) differs from the bacterial populations found in the gingival sulci, tongue, or on the mucous membranes.

Microorganisms entering the mouth first make contact with the saliva or salivary coated surfaces and only those bacteria with adherence capability will be able to be retained. Many of the indigenous bacterial species preferentially colonize specific anatomical locations because their adherence capabilities and complex growth requirements are met. As environmental conditions change, either because of changes in the host or in the microflora itself, the organisms must adapt or be superseded by new species best suited to survive in the new microenvironments. This phenomenon is termed *bacterial succession* and it has great importance in the pathogenesis of many oral infections.

The main environmental selection forces that serve to select the normal oral flora into distinct ecosystems are the anaerobic nature of the oral mucous membranes, the available nutrient sources, and the ability to adhere and survive in the particular niche.

Host-bacterial interrelationships

The interrelationships between the host and the oral microflora are very dynamic. In a healthy state there is a balance between the host defenses and the indigenous microflora. This balance may be broken by an abnormal growth of microorganisms or when there is a decrease in the host defense. The members of the indigenous flora can prevent the colonization of overt pathogens and stimulate the immune system of the host, but these microorganisms may also become pathogenic if allowed to overwhelm or circumvent the host-defense mechanisms. Infections in the oral cavity are usually of this kind. They occur at the microbe's usual anatomical habitat and increase in frequency and severity when other predisposing factors, such as host-debilitating, stress-immune, and nutritional conditions occur.

Dental caries

Dental caries is a slow decomposition of teeth resulting from the loss of hydroxyapatite crystals, which leads to reduced structural integrity of teeth. It is a bacterial infection in which the susceptible tissue is the tooth and the infectious agents are members of the indigenous oral microflora. The carious lesion develops as a result of a change in the ecosystem at the tooth surface, creating a shift in the composition of the microbial flora. The major environmental factor responsible for the development of a cariogenic plaque is diet. An appropriate interaction of plaque bacteria, diet components, host factors, and time is necessary for caries development. Caries occurs when all the aforementioned factors are operating together.

The most consistently found organisms in this lesion are the gram-positive facultative cocci, specifically *Streptococcus mutans* and *Streptococcus salivarius*. *S. mutans* *is the primary etiologic organism in the formation of the carious lesion.* It has the capability of fermenting sugar to lactic acid, which is thought to be responsible for dissolution of the enamel matrix. It also produces great quantities of insoluble extracellular polysaccharides, which allow bacteria to stick to the tooth surface and serve as substrates for energy and acid production. The rapid growth of the streptococci changes factors such as pH, nutrients, and oxidation-reduction potential at the plaque matrix favoring the growth of organisms able to survive under these ecologic conditions (cariogenic plaque). This accumulated plaque is very important in preventing a buffering action of the saliva and thus maintaining the low pH in contact with the tooth surface.

There are three types of dental caries: enamel, dentin, and root surface caries. Enamel surface caries can be further divided into smooth-surface caries and pit and fissure caries. Pit and fissure caries comprise the greatest portion of human lesions. Of the several species of bacteria isolated from these lesions, *S. mutans* is the main etiologic microorganism. *Lactobacillus* sp. are successional bacteria that perpetuate the carious lesion once it is initiated. Dentinal caries exhibit a somewhat different microbial ecology. The organisms at this location must grow in a more anaerobic environment with most of their food source derived from the tooth itself. The most commonly found pathogen at these lesions are lactobacilli. However, other gram-positive anaerobic rods and filaments such as *Bifidobacterium*, *Eubacterium*, and *Propionibacterium* have been identified. The root surface lesion is also associated with a particular microbial ecology. This lesion is initiated on cementum, with a different flora than in smooth-surface lesions, dominated with high numbers of *Actinomyces* sp., although *Lactobacillus* and *S. mutans* have also been identified.

Periodontal disease

The term periodontal disease describes a number of distinct clinical entities that affect the periodontium, including the gingiva, gingival attachment, periodontal ligament, cementum, and supporting alveolar bone. They are all chronic bacterial infections caused by bacteria from dental plaque (see **Table 2.2**). *Like other infections, the bacterial-host interactions determine the nature of the resulting disease.* The pathologic microorganisms may produce disease indirectly, through the effect of toxins, or by direct bacterial invasion of the tissues. The host response to microorganisms may be protective or destructive or both, which accounts for the wide variety of patterns of tissue changes observed in different patients. Periodontal diseases may be generalized or site-specific, may affect different age groups, and may have different rates of progression.

Gingivitis

Gingivitis is defined by chronic inflammation of the gingiva, characterized clinically by changes in color, form, position, and surface appearance. In some instances bleeding and exudate from the gingival sulcus or a pocket may occur.

Experimental gingivitis studies have demonstrated that plaque accumulation at the gingival margin would always produce inflammatory changes in the gingiva. These clinical changes correlate with growth in plaque mass, with the sequential accumulation of different microorganisms (bacterial succession), and with pathological changes at the base of the sulcus. During plaque accumulation, gram-positive rods, specifically *Actinomyces viscosus* and *Actinomyces israelii*, increase proportionally at the expense of gram-positive cocci, and with the formation of an established gingivitis gram-negative bacteria, such as *Fusobacterium, Veillonella, Bacteroides*, and *Treponema* sp., become established.

The composition of the flora associated with gingivitis varies in specific clinical conditions. In pregnancy gingivitis, there are increased proportions of *Bacteroides intermedius* and *Capnocytophaga*, these levels being associated with increased plasma levels of estrogens and progesterone (see chapter 19). In acute necrotizing ulcerative gingivitis (ANUG), the microflora is comprised mainly of fusiform bacilli and spirochetes, with high numbers of *B. intermedius, Selenomonas, Fusobacterium*, and *Treponema* sp.

Periodontitis

Periodontitis occurs by the extension of inflammation and the infection lesion into the deeper structures of the periodontium. Pocket formation, periodontal attachment loss, bone loss, and tooth mobility are the usual clinical features. Periodontal destruction occurs in short periods (burst of activity) followed by periods of quiescence. The resultant anatomical alterations (periodontal pockets) and exposure of furcations create an ecological environment that facilitates the growth of the most pathogenic species and thus facilitates the frequency and duration of episodes of periodontal tissue breakdown.

It is now recognized that several different forms of periodontitis can be distinguished in humans (see **Table 2.2**). These distinct clinical entities have different bacterial profiles and progress and respond differently to a given therapy.

Adult periodontitis is the most common form of periodontitis. It affects adults (35

Table 2.2   Classification of periodontal diseases*

Gingivitis

1. Plaque-associated gingivitis
2. Acute necrotizing ulcerative gingivitis
3. Steroid hormone–influenced gingivitis
4. Medication-influenced gingival overgrowth
5. Desquamative gingivitis

Periodontitis

I.   Adult periodontitis

II. Early-onset periodontitis
     A. Prepubertal periodontitis
        1. Generalized
        2. Localized
     B. Juvenile periodontitis
        1. Generalized
        2. Localized
     C. Rapidly progressive periodontitis

III. Periodontitis associated with systemic disease

IV. Necrotizing ulcerative periodontitis

V.   Refractory periodontitis

---

*Based on the World Workshop in Clinical Periodontics, American Academy of Periodontology, 1989.

years and older). It is usually associated with the presence of large amounts of plaque and calculus and with periodontal attachment loss. Most patients usually do not present evidence of predisposing systemic diseases.

The subgingival microflora in periodontitis is a very complex microbiota with elevated proportions of motile, gram-negative, capnophilic, and anaerobic species (see **Table 2.3**). There are specific microorganisms that appear to be more strongly associated with these lesions: *Bacteroides gingivalis, B. intermedius, Bacteroides forsythus, Bacteroides capillus, Eikenella corrodens, Wolinella recta, Selenomonas sputigena, Eubacterium timidum, Eubacterium brachyi, Eubacterium nodatum, Peptostreptococcus micros, Fusobacterium nucleatum, Actinobacillus* sp., and spirochetes.

Juvenile periodontitis   This disease of the periodontium is characterized by rapid destruction of the periodontal tissues around more than one tooth in the permanent dentition. These lesions progress rapidly after onset but tend to slow with time. The age of onset is circumpubertal, and it is usually manifested in a localized form around incisors and first molars. Clinically, the amount of plaque and calculus is usually minimal in early cases. The subgingival microflora in this disease is predominantly facultative anaerobic gram-negative rods, including *Actinobacillus actinomycetem-*

Table 2.3 Bacteriology of periodontitis

Clinical condition	Associated pathogens
Adult periodontitis	Bacteroides intermedius, Bacteroides gingivalis, Bacteroides capillosus, Eikenella corrodens, Wolinella recta, Eubacterium brachy, Eubacterium timidum, Selenomonas sputigena, Peptostreptococcus micros, Fusobacterium nucleatum, spirochetes
Prepubertal periodontitis	Actinobacillus actinomycetemcomitans, E. corrodens, Capnocytophaga sputigena
Juvenile periodontitis	A. actinomycetemcomitans, E. corrodens, Capnocytophaga sp.
Rapidly progressive periodontitis	B. gingivalis, Bacteroides forsythus, B. intermedius, B. capillosus, E. corrodens, W. recta, A. actinomycetemcomitans
Refractory periodontitis	B. gingivalis, B. forsythus, B. intermedius, A. actinomycetemcomitans, S. intermedius, P. micros

comitans as the most frequently isolated species. However, other subgingival periodontal pathogens usually found in adult periodontitis have also been isolated in this condition. *A. actinomycetemcomitans* presence has been correlated with attachment loss in patients with this disease, and this organism has shown the capability to invade periodontal tissues. In juvenile periodontitis patients, a genetically transmitted functional defect in neutrophil leukocytes has been demonstrated.

Prepubertal periodontitis This condition has its onset during or immediately following eruption of primary teeth. In these children a very severe and rapid periodontal destruction occurs around the primary teeth. Although very rare, it normally occurs as a generalized form and these patients usually present severe defects in their leukocyte and monocyte function that leads to frequent systemic infections. *A. actinomycetemcomitans* is also the most prevalent bacteria found in these lesions.

Rapidly progressive periodontitis This condition affects young adults (20 to 35 years of age) with a generalized severe and rapid periodontal attachment loss. In these patients, the amount of plaque, calculus, and gingival inflammation is low but attachment loss is usually very severe. Some patients have associated host-defense abnormalities. The microflora associated with these lesions is characterized with different associations of the most pathogenic periodontopathic organisms: *B. gingivalis, B. forsythus, B. intermedius, A. actinomycetemcomitans, E. corrodens,* and *W. recta.*

Refractory adult periodontitis This refers to periodontal lesions or patients that are refractory (unresponsive) to periodontal treatment. Different associations of *B. gingivalis, B. forsythus, S. intermedius, B. intermedius,* and *A. actinomycetemcomitans* have been identified with these nonresponding lesions.

Periodontitis associated with HIV-infections   In 1988 two specific periodontal conditions were described associated with HIV-infections: HIV-gingivitis and HIV-periodontitis. HIV-gingivitis is characterized by lesions confined to soft tissues showing distinctive erythema of the free gingiva, attached gingiva, and alveolar mucosa. Spontaneous bleeding is also a consistent finding. Unlike gingivitis, these lesions do not respond to conventional periodontal therapy.

HIV-periodontitis is characterized by severe soft-tissue necrosis and rapid destruction of periodontal attachment and bone; however, affected areas do not show formation of deep pockets. Pain is also a distinguishing feature of HIV-periodontitis, described by patients as being located in the jaws.

HIV-gingivitis and HIV-periodontitis sites have shown high numbers of periodontal pathogens, not different from periodontitis sites in non-HIV patients.

Endodontic and periapical infections (see chapter 12)

Bacteria can gain access to the root canal system in a number of ways:

1. Direct extension through deep carious lesions. Bacterial penetration of the pulp results in an inflammatory response with accumulation of polymorphonuclear neutrophil leukocytes (PMNs) and formation of a pulpal abscess and tissue necrosis.
2. Pulpal injury may result from the local disruption of the pulp's blood supply. The subsequent necrosis of the pulpal tissue represents an ideal environment for colonization and proliferation of anaerobic bacteria.
3. Retrogenic invasion. The pulp may also become injured by retrogenic microbial invasion from diseased periodontal tissues through accessory or lateral canals adjacent to a deep periodontal pocket.

Periapical lesions produce the same progressive changes that occur in the pulp. Depending on the resistance of the host and the number and virulence of invading bacteria, the inflammatory reaction may be acute or chronic and the process may be arrested at any time. Infection always follows the path of least resistance, and normally, a chronic draining sinus tract to the oral cavity develops. Less frequently, the exudate rapidly extends along facial planes to involve other vital tissues or organs, providing an immediate threat to the host.

Infections of odontogenic origin usually harbor a mixed flora with a predominance of anaerobic bacteria, mainly *Bacteroides, Fusobacterium, Peptococcus, Peptostreptococcus, Propionibacterium*, and *Actinomyces* sp.

Progressive infections (see chapter 13)

Progressive mandibular infections can extend through the submandibular, sublingual, and submental spaces, the floor of the mouth, and the upper cervical areas. These infections are characterized by a rapidly spreading indurated cellulitis that may cause edema of the pharynx and strangulation. Extension of maxillary infections can also result in critical conditions. Cellulitis and abscesses may extend into the orbit or may affect the cavernous sinus. Most of the bacteria recovered from these space infections belong to the same anaerobic species as those described for endodontic infections and periodontal diseases.

Further reading

Caton, J. 1987. Periodontal diagnosis and diagnostic aids. In *Proceedings of the World Workshop in Clinical Periodontics*. Chicago: American Academy of Periodontology.

Newman, M.G., and Sanz, M. 1987. Oral microbiology with emphasis on etiology. In *Perspectives on Oral Antimicrobial Therapeutics*. Chicago: American Academy of Periodontology.

Nisengard R.J., Newman, M.G., and Zambon, J.J. 1988. Periodontal diseases. *In* Newman, M.G., and Nisengard, R.J. (eds.) *Oral Microbiology and Immunology*. Philadelphia: W.B. Saunders Co.

Sanz, M., and Newman, M.G. 1988. Dental plaque and calculus. *In* Newman, M.G., and Nisengard, R.J. (eds.) *Oral Microbiology and Immunology*. Philadelphia: W.B. Saunders Co.

Sanz, M., Newman, M.G., and Nisengard, R.J. 1990. Microbiology of periodontal diseases. *In* Carranza, F.A. (ed.) *Clinical Periodontology*. 7th ed. Philadelphia: W.B. Saunders Co.

Wolinsky, L.E. 1988. Caries and cariology. *In* Newman, M.G., and Nisengard, R.J. (eds.) *Oral Microbiology and Immunology*. Philadelphia: W.B. Saunders Co.

PART 2

DRUGS OF CHOICE

CHAPTER 3

Testing Antimicrobial Susceptibility

Sushma Nachnani, M.S.
Michael G. Newman, D.D.S.

In dentistry, many oral infections are successfully treated empirically without identification or knowledge of the specific etiologic agent. This approach is not always correct because unsuspected resistance can occur, resulting in unsuccessful or inadequate treatment. In situations where susceptibility tests are indicated, the nature of the test and the subsequent interpretations are critical for an optimum therapeutic result (see **Table 3.1**).

Because of bacterial resistance, a major role is played by the bacteriology laboratory in performing the in vitro sensitivity tests. These tests are essential for determining a microorganism's sensitivity or resistance to a particular agent used in therapy.

When resistance develops during a course of treatment, it may deprive the host of a complete or optimum therapeutic effect. The elimination of sensitive strains and the dissemination of resistant ones lead to a situation in the population in which many infections become resistant to normal therapy; alternative treatment must then be adopted. For example, penicillin has traditionally been the recommended chemotherapy for most infections involving black-pigmented *Bacteroides*. However, recent studies have suggested that over time, increasing resistance of this organism has developed to penicillin and to other commonly prescribed antibiotics.[1-6] In addition, some microorganisms produce enzymes that inactivate penicillin, cephalosporins, and

Table 3.1 When antibiotic susceptibility tests should be recommended

Oral surgery	Acute infection; septicemia
Endodontics	Endodontal abscess; diffuse and/or unresponsive infection
Periodontics	Refractory cases; relapsing or recurrent infection
Implant therapy	Incomplete wound healing; peri-implant infection

aminoglycosides. Bacteria that produce penicillinase have been shown to inactivate penicillin in vivo in animal models.[7,8] Purulent exudates can also inactivate penicillin.[9,10]

Antibiotic susceptibility tests are intended to be a guide for the clinician, not a guarantee that an antimicrobial agent will be effective in therapy (see **Table 3.1**). The clinician must make the final choice based on his or her knowledge of the pertinent facts of the particular case. This includes knowledge of the infectious agent, its susceptibility, the pharmacology of the drugs being considered, and details about the patient's medical and dental history.

Limitations to in vitro tests

Laboratory results can only give an indication of what the clinical activity of the drug will be. The effect of the drug in vivo depends on: *(1)* its ability to reach the site of infection in a high enough concentration to inhibit the pathogen; *(2)* the nature of the pathological process; and *(3)* the immune response of the host.

Measuring inhibition by drugs

Types of data   The actions of antibiotics or chemotherapeutic agents against pathogenic or potentially pathogenic microorganisms can be measured qualitatively, semiquantitatively, or quantitatively.

Qualitative degrees of susceptibility

Susceptible   A microorganism is regarded as *susceptible* if it is inhibited by a concentration of an antimicrobial agent that is less than that obtained in the blood or tissues of patients treated with doses recommended for the type of infection and type of microorganism involved.

Resistant   A microorganism is regarded as *resistant* if concentrations of the antimicrobial agent required for inhibition are about those ordinarily obtained in the blood or in the tissues during therapy. A strain is resistant if it can tolerate antibiotic concentrations considerably higher than the concentrations that inhibit most other strains in the same species.

Intermediate   A small group of organisms are termed *intermediate* in their susceptibility of an antimicrobial agent if the inhibitory concentration is equal to or slightly higher than that normally obtained in the blood with normal dosages.

Quantitative tests

A quantitative test determines how much the minimal inhibitory concentration inhibits growth of the organism.

MIC   The lowest concentration of the agent that inhibits the growth of the organism, as detected by lack of visual turbidity, is designated the *minimum inhibitory concentration* (MIC).

MBC or MLC   The lowest concentration of antimicrobial agent that allows less than 0.1% of the original inoculum to survive is said to be the *minimum bactericidal concentration* (MBC), also called the *minimum lethal concentration* (MLC).

Special considerations in susceptibility testing

β-lactamases

These heterogenous bacterial enzymes cleave the β-lactam ring of penicillin and cephalosporins to inactivate the antibiotic. They are present on the bacterial chromosome or on plasmids that can be transferred from one bacterium to another. The β-lactamase may be constitutive, or it may be produced only after the bacterium has encountered the antibiotic. Some enzymes predominantly affect penicillins; others affect cephalosporins and still others have broad activity.

The *chromogenic cephalosporin test* employing nitrocephin is a sensitive method to detect the β-lactamase enzyme. Filter paper discs impregnated with nitrocephin are commercially available. In the laboratory, a loopful of a colony is smeared on the disc and placed in a closed petri dish to prevent rapid dessication. Organisms that contain β-lactamase will change the color of the disc from yellow to red. The reaction usually occurs within 30 seconds, but tests are read finally after 15 minutes.

McFarland standard

For all susceptibility testing, a standard inoculum of the bacteria must be used. The number of bacteria in the liquid medium can be determined by counting individual cells in a microscopic counting chamber such as the Petroff Hausser Chamber. This may also be accomplished by measuring the optical density of the broth culture containing the bacteria (stationary phase) to a standard that represents a known number of bacteria in suspension. Those so-called turbidity standards can be prepared by mixing chemical solutions that precipitate to form a solution of reproducible turbidity. Such solutions consisting of barium sulfate and sulfuric acid were developed by McFarland[11] to

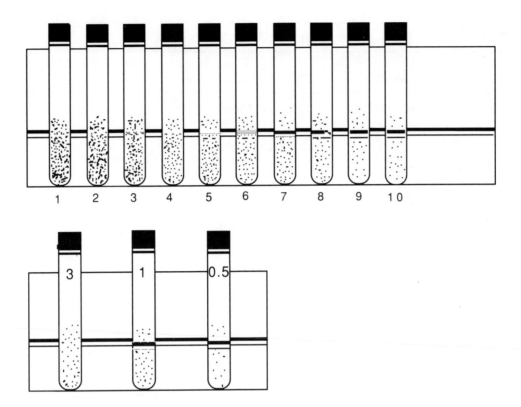

Fig. 3.1 McFarland Standard: *(top)* serial dilutions of test bacteria; *(below)* visual comparison of the turbidity of the liquid medium to a standard that represents a known number of bacteria in suspension. The tubes are held against a paper with a bold line drawn on it. A 0.5 McFarland Standard is used for all susceptibility testing.

approximate numbers of bacteria to solutions of equal turbidity, as determined by colony counts (see **Fig. 3.1**).

Methods of susceptibility testing

Factors influencing results

Results of susceptibility tests are influenced greatly by the reagents and the conditions of the tests (see **Table 3.2**).

Inoculum Inoculum, size, and density are especially critical. It is important that the

---

Table 3.2 Factors affecting susceptibility test results

Type of test	Variable factor
Dilution and diffusion	Inoculum preparation
	Medium
	pH
	Atmosphere of incubation
	Incubation time and temperature
	Stability of antimicrobial agent
Diffusion	Disc content
	Medium depth
	Prediffusion time

---

inoculum be derived from several colonies of the organism to be tested. This is done to reduce the chance of selecting variants more susceptible than the majority of the organisms in the population. This also increases the chance of including representatives of more resistant organisms in a population heterogenous in its susceptibility. For some combinations of bacteria and antibiotic, the inoculum is important in determining the in vitro susceptibility.[12,13] Enzymatic inactivation of β-lactam antibiotics, such as the penicillins and the cephalosporins, is an important mechanism of bacterial resistance. These enzymes are always expressed in some bacteria but must be induced by the presence of the antibiotic in other bacteria. If small numbers of *Staphylococcus aureus*, which contain an inducible β-lactamase, are incubated in vitro with penicillin, the bacteria may be killed before the enzyme can be produced in effective quantities. In contrast, large numbers of bacteria in an active clinical infection may survive to produce the inactivating enzyme and destroy the antibiotic. In this case, a false impression of bacterial susceptibility and a false sense of security might be produced by the laboratory test.

Ph   Antimicrobial susceptibility tests are standardized at physiologic pH at 7.2 to 7.4, yet nonphysiologic levels of pH often develop at the site of purulent infections such as bacterial meningitis[14] or abscesses.[15] Some antibiotics such as penicillins and cephalosporins function well at a wide range of pH. Tetracyclines function better in more acidic environments. In contrast, aminoglycosides and macrolides, such as erythromycin, are less effective in acidic environments than at neutral pH.

Cations   With certain combinations of bacteria and antibiotics, most notably *Pseudomonas aeruginosa* and aminoglycosides, the concentration of divalent cations, particularly calcium and magnesium, has a dramatic effect on the apparent in vitro susceptibility. A result that ranges from susceptible to resistant can be achieved by varying the cation concentration.[16] Agar and broth media vary greatly in the concentration of divalent cations. By convention, testing is done under physiologic conditions. The concentration of calcium and magnesium should be 10 to 12.5 mg/L and 20 to 25 mg/L, respectively.

Medium   Variation in medium composition can influence results with many antimicrobial agents. The inactivation of sulfonamides by para-aminobenzoic acid in some culture media has long been recognized. Thymidine reduces the antibacterial effect of sulfonamides and trimethoprim. Calcium, magnesium, and other metallic cations in media bind to tetracycline and reduce its activity. Calcium and magnesium also affect the permeability of *Pseudomonas* cell membranes to gentamicin, and strains appear more resistant with increasing concentrations of these ions. Acidic media enhances the actions of some antimicrobials (tetracycline, methicillin, and novobiocin) or inhibits others (aminoglycosides, macrolides, and lincomycins).

Incubation   An anaerobic atmosphere appears to affect the permeability of aminoglycosides; CO_2 lowers the pH of the medium to increase or decrease the activity of various drugs as indicated above.

Prolonged incubation usually results in higher minimal inhibitory concentrations in dilution tests or smaller zones of inhibition in diffusion tests. This effect is usually more pronounced with bacteriostatic drugs and with drugs that are unstable at the incubation temperature used.

Antibiotic diffusion   The zones of inhibited growth surrounding the discs depend on the diffusion of the antibiotic into the medium during the period between application of inoculum and initiation of organism growth. Diffusion can vary with amount of antibiotic in the disc, depth of the medium, and whether time is allowed for diffusion before incubation of the test.

Temperature   Plates and tubes should be incubated routinely at 35°C.

Quality control   Rigorous quality control is important for antimicrobial susceptibility testing because of the large number of variables that may affect the results. Some of the physical and chemical characteristics of the media, such as pH and depth of the agar, may be monitored, but the final control is provided by a series of reference bacterial strains for which expected results have been established. These reference strains are available from the American Type Culture Collection in Washington, D.C., or from various commercial sources.

Disc diffusion method

A variety of laboratory techniques can be used to measure the individual susceptibility of bacteria to antimicrobial agents. Reliable results can be obtained with the **disc diffusion test**. This approach uses a standardized methodology that incorporates the measurement of zone diameters representing the ability of a particular agent to exert its effect. It is correlated with the minimal inhibitory concentration and the behavior of standard strains' known sensitivity and resistance. Methods based solely on the presence or absence of zones of inhibition without regard to size of the zone are not acceptable. The standardized method currently recommended by the National Committee for Clinical Laboratory Standards (NCCLS)[17] subcommittee on antimicrobial susceptibility tests is based on methods described by Bauer et al.[18] It consists of placing filter paper discs containing a fixed amount of antimicrobial on the agar plate, which has been streaked with standard inoculum of the bacteria. After the agar plates have been incubated, the zones of incubation are measured and interpreted according to the committee's established standards (see **Fig. 3.2**). The zones should be measured against a black background and should be differentiated from hemolysis or discoloration of media. The procedure has wide application because the disc can carry most antimicrobial agents. Diffusion tests provide qualitative results, defining organisms as susceptible, intermediate, or resistant to a specific agent.

Although technically simple, the disc diffusion method requires careful attention to detail. *Failure to carefully adhere to the FDA-NCCLS standards, which are based on detailed clinical studies, can yield misleading results.* Standard criteria for several drugs and types of bacteria are given by Barry and Thornsberry[19] and by the NCCLS.

There is presently no consensus on the condition for susceptibility testings of strictly anaerobic organisms, although much work is presently in progress. One such approach offers promise as a rapid resistance screening method. With this method, the antimicrobial susceptibility was compared with the broth dilution method for *Bacteroides intermedius*, which is a suspected periodontopathic microorganism. In the rapid resistance method, the antibiotic discs were placed on trypticase soy agar plates supplemented with 5% rabbit blood incubated with a *mixed culture from the original dental plaque sample*, including facultative and obligate anaerobes. The results are encouraging because the percentage of agreement compared to broth dilution was 88%

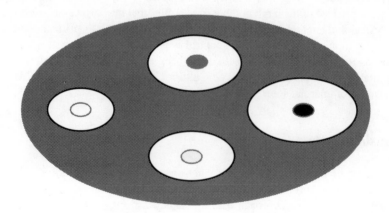

Fig. 3.2   Measuring zones of inhibition on a disc diffusion susceptibility test plate. The diameter of the zone increases with the concentration of the antibiotic on the disc.

to 100% for six different antibiotics studied.[20] If validated further, this method may be used to provide a rapid mechanism for determining general susceptibility profiles for the clinician.

Limitations   The above disc methods have been standardized for testing rapidly growing pathogens, such as *Enterobacteriaceae, Staphylococcus* sp., and *Pseudomonas* sp., and for some antibiotics with *Haemophilus* sp., *Neisseria* sp., and *Streptococcus pneumoniae*. Studies are not yet adequate to develop reproducible definitive standards for interpretation of disc tests with other microorganisms *that cause oral infections and require an anaerobic atmosphere*. These organisms demonstrate a poor or slow growth rate on Mueller-Hinton agar or manifest marked strain-to-strain variations in the rate of growth.

Standardizations of the disc diffusion test for the oral microbiota and anaerobic bacteria of medical importance have been attempted,[21,22] but these are not officially accepted.

Dilution methods

Macrodilution test   The most *quantitative* way to test antimicrobial susceptibility is to use one of the dilution tests recommended by the International Collaborative Study[23] or the NCCLS.[24] These avoid some of the problems encountered with the diffusion properties of antimicrobials discussed above. A dilution test does not have the flexibility of a diffusion test, however. When results are reported quantitatively, the clinician must know individual drug pharmacology.

Dilution tests are generally performed by preparing a series of two-fold serial dilutions of an antimicrobial agent in a nutrient medium, either liquid or solid (see **Fig. 3.3**). These are inoculated with a standardized culture of the organism and incubated in an appropriate atmosphere. The concentration of drug that inhibits growth is then determined.

If the test has been performed in a liquid medium, subcultures can be made from tubes showing inhibition to determine the lethal (bactericidal) concentration. The tube that shows no growth or barely visible growth is the MBC. Lennette and coworkers[25] described standard procedures for broth and agar dilution and microdilution tests for all types of bacteria.

Simplified versions of broth and agar dilution procedures using selected concentrations of antimicrobial agents to cover the complete range of susceptibility have been found useful in many laboratories.[26-28]

Broth disc or disc tube method   One of the simplest modifications of the standard antimicrobial susceptibility methods has been the disc tube method first described by Schneiersen[29] and later adapted for use with anaerobes and spirochetes.[30-33] In this method one or more discs are added to the medium appropriate for growth of the organism to be tested. The antibiotic elutes from the discs to give the desired concentration of the media.

53

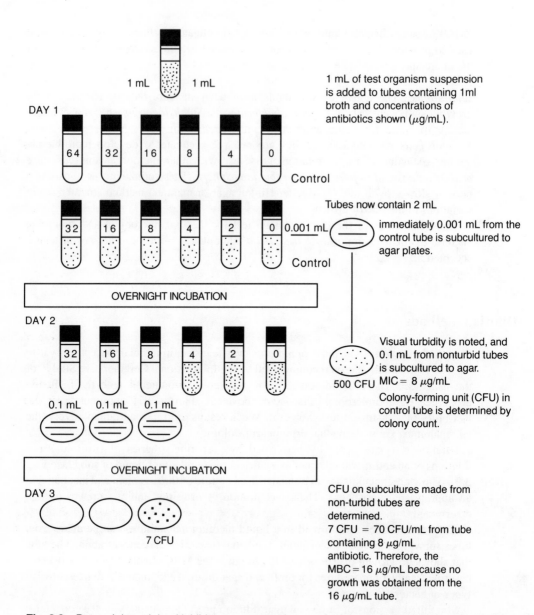

Fig. 3.3 Determining minimal inhibitory concentrations and minimum bactericidal concentration.

Microdilution method   Microdilution tests are miniaturized variations of the broth dilution procedure. Plastic trays containing eight or more rows of small, flat-bottomed U- or V-shaped wells are used. Special calibrated loops are used for making antibiotic dilution and inoculating the bacteria; 50 μL of the dilutions of the various antibiotics are added to each well and the series of serial dilutions are made in each row.

The inoculum is grown in the same manner as described above (0.5 McFarland Standard). In each well 50 μL of the inoculum is added and the plates are incubated for 48 hours anaerobically. The MIC is read as the lowest concentration of drug showing no visible growth.

Agar dilution method   Agar dilution tests are convenient when large numbers of strains are to be tested or when broth growth is unpredictable. Test results are often easier to read and there is the advantage of visual detection of contaminants. Dilutions of drugs are prepared and incorporated into agar. The turbidity of the inoculum is adjusted to 0.5 McFarland Standard and applied to the plates by means of Steer's-Foltz replicator (Graft Machine Inc., Chester, Pa.) (see **Fig. 3.4**). The "Steer's" replicator has 32 wells for the inoculum; one can use this machine to stamp many plates of different dilutions of the antibiotic. One plate without the antibiotic is incubated as a negative control. Strains of known susceptibility are incubated as a positive control. After the plates have been incubated, the MIC is read as the lowest concentration of drug yielding no growth.

Clinical indications   Dilution tests are recommended for the slow-growing facultative anaerobic bacteria found in oral infections, as well as for fungi. Dilution methods also determine bactericidal activity or evidence of synergism or antagonism between antimicrobial agents against particular bacteria.

Interpretation of results

The susceptibility of an isolate will be reported as the MIC (see **Tables 3.3** and **3.4**). Interpretation requires information about the levels of the agent that can be achieved in a patient's blood or tissues. In general, an organism is considered susceptible if the MIC is substantially lower than the peak concentration in the blood.

Peak serum concentrations of several antimicrobial agents are shown in **Table 3.5**; see chapter 5 for additional prescribing information.

Using test results

Selection of an antimicrobial agent, dosage schedule, and administration route is based on the considerations as shown in **Table 3.6**.

Susceptibility tests may need to be supplemented with other procedures in certain complex situations, especially subacute bacterial endocarditis and in severe infections.

An example of a laboratory report form used to guide the treatment of patients in refractory periodontitis is shown in **Fig. 3.5**. The culture isolation and antibiotic testing

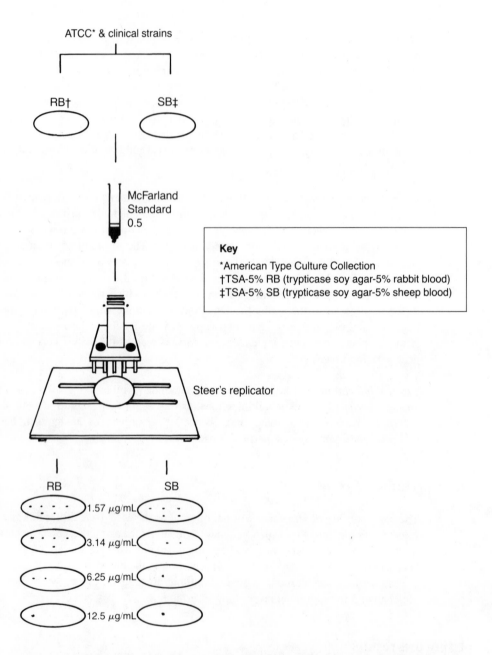

Fig. 3.4   An aliquot of the organism to be tested is diluted to 0.5 McFarland Standard. Each aliquot is placed into one well of the replicating inoculator device. This device has metal prongs that are calibrated to pick up a small amount of bacterial suspension (usually 0.001 μL), which is delivered to a series of agar plates.

Table 3.3 Minimum inhibitory concentrations for 90% of anaerobic isolates*

MIC†

Antimicrobial agent	Black-pigmented Bacteroides (40)‡		Fusobacterium (13)		Other gram-negative bacilli (13)§		Veillonella (8)		Gram-positive cocci (11)		Eubacterium (7)	
	Range	90%	Range	90%	Range	90%	Range	90%	Range	90%	Range	90%
Penicillin G	≤0.06–64	0.5	≤0.06–8	0.5	≤0.06–32	4	0.25–0.5	0.5	≤0.06–0.5	0.25	≤0.06–0.5	0.5
Cefadroxil	≤0.06–128	4	0.25–16	8	0.25–64	64	≤0.06–1	0.5	≤0.06–64	16	0.13–64	4
Cephalexin	0.5–32	2	0.5–8	8	0.5–16	16	0.25–1	0.5	0.13–32	8	0.25–64	4
Cephradine	0.25–32	2	0.5–8	8	0.5–32	32	0.13–0.5	0.25	0.5–128	32	0.5–64	16
Cefoperazone	0.13–8	2	≤0.06–8	1	0.25–128	32	0.25–2	2	≤0.06–1	1	≤0.06–2	1
Moxalactam	≤0.06–32	1	0.25–16	16	≤0.06–16	8	≤0.06–2	1	≤0.06–4	2	≤0.06–8	0.5
Sch 29,482	≤0.06–2	0.13	≤0.06–1	1	≤0.06–1	0.5	0.13–0.5	0.25	≤0.06–1	0.5	≤0.06–0.25	0.25
Clindamycin	≤0.06–0.5	0.13	≤0.06–0.25	0.25	≤0.06–2	1	≤0.6–0.25	0.25	≤0.06–0.5	0.5	≤0.06–2	1
Erythromycin	0.13–>128	1	0.5–128	128	≤0.06–2	2	16–64	64	≤0.06–2	2	≤0.06–0.25	0.25
Metronidazole	≤0.06–32	1	≤0.06–0.25	0.25	≤0.06–2	2	0.5–1	1	≤0.06–2	2	≤0.06–64	64
Tetracycline	≤0.06–16	2	≤0.06–16	1	≤0.06–16	1	0.5–2	2	≤0.06–2	1	≤0.06–4	1
Colistin	0.5–>128	>128	0.25–2	1	≤0.06–>128	>128	1–2	1	32–>128	>128	8–>128	>128
Kanamycin	8–>128	>128	0.5–>128	128	0.5–>128	>128	32–>128	64	0.5–>128	128	4–>128	>128
Vancomycin	4–>128	128	16–>128	>128	1–>128	>128	32–>128	>128	0.13–1	1	0.5–2	1

*Source: Sutter et al. (1983).[34] Reprinted by permission from the American Society for Microbiology.
†Minimal inhibitory concentrations are expressed in micrograms per milliliter, except penicillin G, which is expressed in units per milliliter. Numbers in parentheses indicate number of strains tested. 90%, MIC inhibiting 90% of isolates.
‡Includes *Bacteroides melaninogenicus, Bacteroides loeschii, Bacteroides denticola, Bacteroides intermedius, Bacteroides corporis, Bacteroides asaccharolyticus, Bacteroides gingivalis,* and the type strain of *Bacteroides macacae.*
§Includes *Bacteroides oralis, Bacteroides ureolyticus,* other *Bacteroides* sp., *Selenomonas* sp., and *Wolinella* sp.

Table 3.4   Minimum inhibitory concentrations for 90% of selected oral isolates*
Microaerophilic and facultative isolates only

MIC†

Antimicrobial agent	Capnocytophaga (17)		Eikenella and Haemophilus (2)‡		Actinomyces (22)§		Arachnia and Propionibacterium (6)§		Lactobacillus (16)§		Streptococcus (39)	
	Range	90%	Range	90%	Range	90%	Range	90%	Range	90%	Range	90%
Penicillin G	0.25–1	1	0.25–0.5	0.5	≤0.06–8	1	≤0.06–0.13	0.13	≤0.06–0.5	0.25	≤0.06–0.5	0.25
Cefadroxil	2–>128	128	8–32	32	≤0.06–2	1	0.13–8	8	≤0.06–1	0.5	0.25–32	16
Cephalexin	1–128	64	4–16	16	≤0.06–2	1	0.25–32	32	≤0.06–2	0.5	0.5–32	16
Cephradine	2–>128	128	8–16	16	0.25–8	4	0.25–64	64	≤0.06–1	1	0.25–32	16
Cefoperazone	0.25–32	8	≤0.06–0.13	0.13	0.13–4	4	0.13–8	8	≤0.06–1	1	≤0.06–4	2
Moxalactam	0.13–16	4	≤0.06	≤0.06	≤0.06–8	4	≤0.06–8	8	0.13–1	0.5	≤0.06–32	8
Sch 29,482	0.25–2	1	0.25–1	1	≤0.06–1	0.5	≤0.06–4	4	≤0.06–0.25	0.25	≤0.06–2	1
Clindamycin	≤0.06–0.13	0.13	16–32	32	≤0.06–4	1	≤0.06–16	16	≤0.06–2	1	≤0.06–128	0.13
Erythromycin	0.13–4	2	1	1	≤0.06–1	0.25	≤0.06–2	2	≤0.06–1	0.5	≤0.06–>128	0.13
Metronidazole	1–32	16	128–>128	>128	0.25–>128	>128	0.5–>128	>128	0.5–>128	>128	128–>128	>128
Tetracycline	0.25–2	2	1	1	0.25–64	4	0.13–2	2	≤0.06–16	1	0.5–128	64
Colistin	128–>128	>128	0.5–1	1	16–>128	>128	128–>128	>128	8–>128	>128	128–>128	>128
Kanamycin	128–>128	>128	1–2	2	8–>128	>128	16–>128	>128	2–128	128	0.5–>128	>128
Vancomycin	0.5–64	32	16–128	128	0.5–8	1	0.25–64	64	0.13–2	1	0.5–2	2

*Source: Sutter et al. (1983).[34] Reprinted by permission from the American Society for Microbiology.
†Concentrations are expressed in micrograms per milliliter, except penicillin G, which is expressed in units per milliliter. Numbers in parentheses indicate number of strains tested. 90%, MIC inhibiting 90% of isolates.
‡One strain each of *Eikenella corrodens* and *Haemophilus aphrophilus*.
§A few strains grew under anaerobic conditions only.

Table 3.5 Peak serum concentrations of antibiotics*

Antimicrobial agent	Route	Serum concentration†
		µg/mL
Penicillins‡	IM/IV	2–200†
Augmentin	Oral	4–7
Benzathine penicillin G	Depot	0.01–0.06
Procaine penicillin G	Depot	0.1–18
Cephalosporins		
Cephalexin	Oral	5–35
Cephadroxyl	Oral	16–28
Cephradine	Oral	5–35
	IV	17–49
Aminoglycosides		
Gentamicin	IV	1–12
Kanamycin	IM	10–25
Streptomycin	IM	10–25
Tetracyclines		
Tetracycline	Oral	1–5
	IV	5–30
Doxycycline	Oral	1–6
Minocycline	Oral	0.7–4.5
Clindamycin	Oral	5–26
Chloramphenicol	Oral	3–12
	IV	20–40
Erythromycin	Oral	<1–10
	IV	5–30
Lincomycin	IV/IM	2–20
Metronidazole	Oral	4–10
Vancomycin	IV	20–50

*Source: Sabath (1980).[35]
†Wide ranges represent the effects of different doses, routes of administration, and preparations. Serum concentrations for oral routes will tend toward the low end of the range given.
‡Penicillins include benzylpenicillin, phenoxymethyl penicillin, amoxicillin, carbenicillin, and cloxacillin.

Table 3.6 Considerations for using antimicrobial susceptibility tests

- Relationship of the minimum inhibitory concentration of the specific isolate to blood level data
- Susceptibility of the specific strain with others of the same species
- Clinical experience with the drug for treating similar infections
- Pharmacokinetic factors, such as the ability of the agent to penetrate to the site of the infection
- Host factors, such as compromised defense

PERIODONTAL MICROBIOLOGY REPORT

Sample # _____

Dr _____   Patient _____

SS # _____

SAMPLE (SITE) INFORMATION

Yes   No

Site _____   Local factors: Bleeding ____ ____
                                                 Suppuration ____ ____
Date collected _____   Restoration ____ ____
            Tooth & location   Other ____ ____

Bacteriology   ## Antimicrobial susceptibility'

Presumptive ID of selective isolates*	Quantity estimate†	P E N	A M P	A U G	T E T	C L I	M E T
A.a‡	+ +	S	S	S	S	S	S
B.P.B.§	+ + +	S	S	S	S	S	S
B. gingivalis	+ + +	S	S	S	S	S	S
B. intermedius							
Wolinella species							
S.T.B.#	+ +	S	S	S	S	R	S
Eikenella corrodens							
Capnocytophaga species							

*Bacteriology results reflect cultivable bacteria at time of laboratory processing.

†ND <10⁴
+   10⁴
+ +   10⁵
+ + +>10⁵

‡A.a. = *Actinobacillus actinomycetemcomitans.*
§B.P.B. = Black-pigmented *Bacteroides* species.
#S.T.B. = Surface translocating bacteria.

¶ Antimicrobial susceptibility:

Drugs tested	Therapeutic dose P.O.	Attainable blood level
Penicillin	250mg qid	1–3µg/mL
Ampicillin	250mg qid	4–6µg/mL
Augmentin	250mg tid	4–6µg/mL
Tetracycline	250mg qid	1–5µg/mL**
Clindamycin	150mg tid	4–5µg/mL
Metronidazole	250mg tid	4–6µg/mL

**May be higher in crevicular fluid.

Fig. 3.5

that are routinely performed in clinical laboratories are too complex, costly, and time-consuming to apply to all periodontal samples. However, in refractory or unusual cases, the development of selective culture media and the streamlining of traditional antibiotic susceptibility testing has allowed some laboratories to offer diagnostic testing services for the presumptive identification and susceptibility testing of periodontal pathogens.

These clinical bacteriology laboratories usually supply interested dental offices with a culture collection kit upon request. All supplies needed for collection and shipping of a periodontal culture are included in this kit.

References

1. Applebaum, P.C., and Chatterton, S.A. 1987. Susceptibility of anaerobic bacteria to ten antimicrobial agents. *Antimicrob. Agents Chemother.* 14:371–376.

2. Brown, W.J., and Waatti, P.E. 1980. Susceptibility testing of clinically isolated anaerobic bacteria by an agar dilution technique. *Antimicrob. Agents Chemother.* 17:629–635.

3. Marrie, T.J., Haldane, E.V., Swantee, C.A., and Kerr, E.A. 1981. Susceptibility to antimicrobial agents and demonstrations of decreased susceptibility of *Clostridium perfringens* to penicillin. *Antimicrob. Agents Chemother.* 19:51–55.

4. Murray, P.R., and Rosenbatt, J.E. 1977. Penicillin resistance and penicillinase production in clinical isolates of *Bacteroides melaninogenicus*. *Antimicrob. Agents Chemother.* 11:605–608.

5. Niederan, W.U., Hoffler, X., and Pulverer, G. 1980. Susceptibility of *Bacteroides melaninogenicus* to 45 antibiotics. *Antimicrob. Agents Chemother.* 26:121–127.

6. Sutter, V.L., and Finegold, S.M. 1976. Susceptibility of anaerobic bacteria to 23 antimicrobial agents. *Antimicrob. Agents Chemother.* 10:736–752.

7. Hackman, A.S., and Wilkins, T.D. 1976. Influence of penicillinase production by strains of *Bacteroides melaninogenicus* and *Bacteroides oralis* on penicillin therapy of an experimental mixed anaerobic infection in mice. *Arch. Oral Biol.* 21:385–398.

8. O'Keefe, J.P., Tally, F.P., Barza, T.M., and Gorbach, S.L. 1978. Inactivation of penicillin G during experimental infection with *Bacteroides fragilis*. *J. Infect. Dis.* 137:437–442.

9. Barnes, P., and Waterworth, P.M. 1977. New cause of penicillin treatment failure. *Br. Med. J.* 1:991–993.

10. deLouvois, J., and Hurley, R. 1977. Inactivation of penicillin by purulent exudates. *Br. Med. J.* 1:998–1000.

11. Sutter, V.L., Citron, D.M., and Finegold, S.M. 1980. *Wadsworth Anaerobic Bacteriology Manual*. 3rd ed. St. Louis: The C.V. Mosby Co., pp. 76–80.

12. Eng, R.H.K., Smith, S.M., Cherubin, C. 1984. Inoculum effect of new β-Lactam antibiotics on *Pseudomonas aeruginosa*. *Antimicrob. Agents Chemother.* 26:42–47.

13. Archer, G.L. 1984. *Staphylococcus epidermidis*: The organism, its diseases, and treatment. *Curr. Clin. Topics Infect. Dis.* 5:25–48.

14. Strausbaugh, L.J., San de, M.A. 1978. Factors influencing the therapy of experimental *Proteus mirabilis* meningitis in rabbits. *J. Infect. Dis.* 137:251–260.

15. Hays, R.C., and Mandell, G.L. 1974. CO_2 pH, redox potential of experimental abscesses. *Proc. Soc. Exp. Biol. Med.* 147:29–30.

16. Relles, L.B., Schoenknecht, F.D., Kenny, M.A., et al. Antibiotic susceptibility testing of *Pseudomonas aeruginosa*: Selection of control strain and criteria for magnesium and calcium content in media. *J. Infect. Dis.* 130:454–463.

17. National Committee for Clinical Laboratory Standards (NCCLS). 1979. Approved Standard ASM-2. *Performance Standards for Antimicrobial Disc Susceptibility Test*. Villanova, Pa.:NCCLS.

18. Bauer, A.W., Kirby, W.M.M., Sherris, J.C., and Turck, M. 1966. Antibiotic susceptibility testing by a standardized simple disc method. *Am. J. Clin. Pathol*. 45:496.

19. Barry, A.L., and Thornsberry, C. 1980. Susceptibility test procedures: Diffusion test procedures. *In* E.H. Lennette et al. (eds.) *Manual of Clinical Microbiology*. 3rd ed. Washington, D.C.: American Society for Microbiology, pp. 463–479.

20. Calsina, G., Lee, Y.S., Newman, M.G., Kornman, K.S., Nachnani, S., and Flemmig, T.F. (In press, 1990.). Rapid antimicrobial resistance screening method for *Bacteroides intermedius*. *Oral Microbiol. Immunol*.

21. Newman, M.G., Hulem, C., Colgate, J., and Anselmo, C. 1979. Antibiotic susceptibility of plaque bacteria. *J. Dent. Res*. 58:1722–1732.

22. Sutter, V.L., Citron, D.M., and Finegold, S.M. 1980. *Wadsworth Anaerobic Bacteriology Manual*. 3rd ed. St. Louis: The C.V. Mosby Co., pp. 76–80.

23. Ericsson, H.M., and Sherris, J.C. 1971. Antibiotic sensitivity testing. Report of an international collaborative study. *Acta. Pathol. Scand*. 217 (Suppl. B):1–90.

24. National Committee for Clinical Laboratory Standards (NCCLS). 1979. Proposed Standard PSM-11. *Proposed Reference Dilution Procedure for Antimicrobial Susceptibility Testing of Anaerobic Bacteria*. Villanova, Pa.:NCCLS.

25. Lennette, E.H., Balows, A., Hausler, W.J., Jr., and Truant, J.P. (eds.) 1980. *Manual of Clinical Microbiology*. 3rd ed. Washington, D.C.: American Society for Microbiology, pp. 446–500.

26. Witebsky, F.G., MacLowry, J.D., and French, S.S. 1979. Broth dilution minimum inhibitory concentrations: Rationale for use of selected antimicrobial concentrations. *J. Clin. Microbiol*. 9:589–595.

27. Hauser, K.J., Johnston, J.A., and Zabransky, R.J. 1975. Economical agar dilution technique for susceptibility testing of anaerobes. *Antimicrob. Agents Chemother*. 7:712–714.

28. Stalons, D.R., and Thornsberry, C. 1975. Broth dilution method for determining the antibiotic susceptibility of anaerobic bacteria. *Antimicrob. Agents Chemother*. 7:15–21.

29. Schneiersen, S.S. 1954. A simple rapid disc-tube method for determination of bacterial sensitivity to antibiotics. *Antibiot. Chemother*. 4:125–132.

30. Alvarez, J.P. 1955. A simplified sensitivity procedure for anaerobic microorganisms. *Am. J. Med. Tech*. 21:249–253.

31. Wilkins, T.D., and Thiel, T. 1973. Modified broth-disk method for testing the antibiotic susceptibility of anaerobic bacteria. *Antimicrob. Agents Chemother*. 3:350–356.

32. Kurzynski, T.A., Yrios, J.W., Helstad, A.G., and Field, C.R. 1976. Aerobically incubated thioglycolate broth disk method for antibiotic susceptibility testing of anaerobes. *Antimicrob. Agents Chemother*. 10:727–732.

33. Abramson, I.J., and Smibert, R.M. 1972. Method for testing antibiotic sensitivity of spirochetes, using antibiotic discs. *Br. J. Vener. Dis*. 48:269–273.

34. Sutter, V.L., Jones, J.M., and Ghoniem, A.T.M. 1983. Antimicrobial susceptibilities of bacteria associated with periodontal disease. *Antimicrob. Agents Chemother*. 23:483–486.

35. Sabath, L.D. 1980. Peak serum concentrations frequently obtained with some antibiotics. *In* E.H. Lennette et al. (ed.) *Manual of Clinical Microbiology*. 3rd ed. Washington, D.C.: American Society of Microbiology. 500:Appendix 3.

CHAPTER 4

Cultural Microbiology Sampling and Analysis

Mariano Sanz, M.D., D.D.S.

The value of testing Effective management of serious, acute, and chronic infections requires laboratory tests to identify the infectious bacteria and their susceptibility. In "refractory" periodontitis patients, microbiology tests are important to guide therapy (see chapter 11). If time is not critical, laboratory tests *before* therapy begins ensure that the antibiotic treatment most specific for the infection is initiated. Quantitative tests (see chapter 3) can be very helpful in determining the antibiotic levels needed in persistent infections.

In the near future, chairside bacteria screening tests will be available. These can be used to guide initial therapy or to monitor therapy rendered.

Obtaining adequate data

The dentist's role in communication Thorough, effective communication between dentist and laboratory personnel is needed to obtain adequate information about the microorganisms present in an infection. The dentist should specify clearly to laboratory personnel which types of organisms to test for (e.g., oral streptococci, aerobic and/or anaerobic pathogens). The dentist also should know and follow the laboratory's requirements for collecting and submitting microbial specimens.

Problems caused by mixed flora The mixed flora usually found in exudates from the soft and osseous orofacial tissues can present technical problems for many hospital bacteriologists, many of whom have little experience diagnosing oral tissue infections. Often they are unaware that in a submucosal or osseous tissue infection culture results should reflect *all* of the bacteria seen in abundance and not just one or two of several major forms present. For example, *Bacteroides* and plaque *Streptococcus* and other facultative oral species are abundant in saliva and would be considered contaminating "normal oral flora" by some hospital microbiology technologists if they detected them in throat samples. Unless advised otherwise, they may also discard such isolates found in specimens taken from the oropharynx. When isolated in large numbers in uncontaminated submucosa and exudates, however, alpha and gamma hemolytic streptococci could be significant pathogens. If concerned about whether these organisms are present in an oral tissue infection, the dentist must specify that their presence be reported.

Laboratory techniques for characterization of oral isolates are available from a wide variety of sources. In addition, several *oral* microbiology testing sources are available that accept specimens from all across the country. Refer to your local periodontist or periodontics department at the most convenient dental school.

Examination of gram-stained direct smears of the exudate should always be requested so that all of the bacteria present in abundance will be reflected.

Testing against specific antibiotics   Tests for the susceptibility of the predominating species should be requested only against specific antibiotics. Without susceptibility test results, the dentist is left to play antibiotic roulette: if the patient does not respond to the first drug selected, the clinician is left to try another almost at random. **The risks are great:** loss of time for recovery, possible exacerbation of the infection, loss of structural tissues, infection of vital organs, hospitalization, and, possibly, loss of life.

Depending on whether the patient responds to initial therapy, the dentist can use susceptibility test results in determining whether to continue the same therapy, change the dosage, or change to a more specific antibacterial therapy.

Guidelines for collecting and submitting specimens

Procedures   When specimens are improperly collected, transported, or submitted, the laboratory may refuse to test them. Most hospital microbiologists will not culture anaerobic exudates from orofacial tissues unless the following criteria are met:

1. Samples for anaerobic culture cannot contain saliva, sputum, gross plaque, or mucosal scrapings. If this is a problem, discuss the situation with the hospital.
2. Samples should be transported according to laboratory specifications, to keep both obligate and facultative anaerobes alive. The proper anaerobic vial or tube should be used and the specimen should be introduced in a manner that will avoid aeration.
3. The correct request forms must be submitted, indicating the important genera suspected whenever possible. Separate exudates must be submitted for aerobic and anaerobic cultures. Separate request forms are sometimes required by a laboratory where aerobes and anaerobes are cultured in separate areas.

Supplies   Sample vials, anaerobic swab tubes, and other supplies noted in the following procedures can be obtained from the laboratory or purchased from local medical supply dealers. They must show expiration dates.

Sampling submucosal lesions

Most laboratories recommend the following procedures. *Bacteriology technicians should be consulted for specific directions.*

Exudate from closed lesions or abscesses   The mucosa is first wiped well with an antiseptic solution (e.g., aqueous iodine or nonphenolic mouthwash) and skin is wiped with iodine and alcohol. Exudate is aspirated with a 20-gauge needle and syringe and injected into an anaerobic transport vial. The anaerobic vial can contain transport medium or may be empty except for a bit of saline. Some laboratories prefer to accept the syringe containing exudate if it can be delivered to the laboratory within 10 minutes.

Exudate from draining lesions or abscesses   When exudates cannot be aspirated, a swab sample of exudate can be collected after the lesion or abscess is incised for drainage. Two methods can be used:

1. A swab from a prereduced tube is used to collect the sample. It is introduced into another prereduced tube and quickly resealed.
2. A swab from an anaerobic pack is used to collect the exudate. The swab is quickly replaced in its pack. Exudates draining from periapical infections through root canals of teeth under endodontic treatment are collected with **absorbent points** (see chapter 12). These are placed in an anaerobic swab transport tube or in a medium provided by the laboratory.

Tissue samples   Procedures for transporting tissue from submucosal lesions are the same as for exudate. If too much air is introduced into the transport tube or vial, the sample must be subcultured in less than 30 minutes or most of the anaerobes will die.

Sampling surface mucosal lesions

After the surface is wiped with a sterile saline-soaked sponge, it is scraped with a split wooden applicator or curette. Mucosal samples need only be submitted for culture of aerobic bacterial pathogens. Anaerobic cultures of mucosal *surface* lesions rarely provide information that cannot be more easily obtained.

Dry smears are prepared on a glass slide for staining (stain for 10 seconds with a 0.1% crystal violet or Gram's stain). Depending on the condition suspected, some direct-access laboratories prefer a wet smear that can first be examined by phase microscopy for fusiforms, motile bacteria, and spirochetes or yeast. The same smear can be stained later for further examination.

Examination for *Actinomyces*

Cultures for *Actinomyces* require a week for incubation and tentative identification.

Requests for cultures of this species should therefore be made only when the clinical condition resembles actinomycosis.

When submitting exudates from a suspected actinomycotic infection, collect as much exudate as possible and place in an anaerobic transport container. Exudates that collect from draining sinus tracts on a gauze bandage should be submitted on the gauze in a well-sealed plastic bag with the request to examine the exudate by Gram's stain for sulfur granules and gram-positive branching rods. Unless it is immediately taken to the laboratory and cultured, such a sample is usually useless for detecting *Actinomyces* sp., even though they are not strictly anaerobic.

Plaque sampling for cariogenic microorganisms

Sampling for cariogenic microorganisms can be carried out from the:

1. Buccolingual smooth surfaces
2. Occlusal surfaces
3. Interproximal surfaces
4. Root surfaces and saliva

Buccolingual smooth surfaces   Small quantities of plaque can be collected by means of a sharp dental instrument, disposable acrylic resin probes, calgi-swabs, and cotton pellets. A sharp dental instrument is recommended because the composition of plaque varies within the thickness of plaque on a tooth surface.

Occlusal surfaces   The most-used method is the wire-scrape method. However, because of the inability to sample into the depth of the pit or fissure, this method may underestimate the load of microorganisms recovered.

Interproximal surfaces   Although a wide variety of sharp dental instruments, needles, abrasive metal strips, and other devices have been used to sample dental plaque, it is not possible to determine whether, in the absence of mechanical separation, the critical subcontact zone has been sampled. For large studies, the dental floss method seems the most suitable.

Root surfaces and saliva   Same as buccolingual smooth surfaces.

Plaque sampling for periodontal microorganisms (see Table 4.1)

In order to take a subgingival plaque for periodontal microorganisms, the sampling device should:

1. Be of a relative size to be introduced in the periodontal pocket in all its length
2. Be able to collect the content of periodontal pocket
3. Not be contaminated by supragingival plaque

Table 4.1 Periodontal conditions when microbial samples and analysis should be recommended

---

I. Adult periodontitis	After conventional periodontal therapy, in unresponsive sites
II. Prepubertal periodontitis	At baseline to check for predominant species and to aid in selection of antimicrobial therapy At different phases of therapy using elimination of predominant species as goal of therapy
III. Juvenile periodontitis	Check for *Actinobacillus actinomycetemcomitans* at the beginning of therapy; use *A. actinomycetemcomitans* elimination as goal of therapy
IV. Rapidly progressing periodontitis	After conventional periodontal therapy, in unresponsive sites to aid in selection of antimicrobial therapy; use elimination of predominant pathogens as goal of therapy
V. Periodontitis associated with systemic diseases	Use elimination of predominant pathogens as goal of therapy
VI. Necrotizing ulcerative periodontitis	After conventional periodontal therapy, in unresponsive sites
VII. Refractory periodontitis	After conventional therapy to aid in selection of antimicrobial therapy; use elimination of predominant pathogens as goal of therapy

---

Various devices have been used for this purpose. The two most currently used devices are the sterile scaler and the sterile paper point. The scaler has the advantage of a higher recovery and of being able to remove both the attached and nonattached component of subgingival plaque. Therefore, it is the most recommended method. However, if subsequent samplings of the same site have to be sampled in short periods of time, the paper point technique is preferred because the scaler tends to deplete the pocket contents. Chapters 2, 3, and 11 are suggested for additional information.

Further reading

Crawford, J.J. 1982. Periapical infections and infections of oral facial tissues. pp. 786–814. *In* J.R. McGhee et al. (eds.) *Dental Microbiology*. New York: Harper & Row.

Holdeman, L.V., Cato, E.P., and Moore, W.E.C. (eds.) 1977. *Anaerobic Laboratory Manual*. 4th ed. Blacksburg, Va.: Virginia Polytechnic Institute and State University.

Keene, H.J. 1986. Sampling of cariogenic microorganisms. *Oral Microbiol. Immunol.* 1:7–13.

Sutter, V.L., Citron, D.M., and Finegold, S.M. 1980. *Wadsworth Anaerobic Bacteriology Manual*: 3rd ed. St. Louis: The C.V. Mosby Co.

Tanner, A.C.R., and Goodson, J.M. 1986. Sampling of microorganisms associated with periodontal disease. *Oral Microbiol. Immunol.* 1:15–21.

CHAPTER 5

Individual Drugs

Mariano Sanz, M.D., D.D.S.
Michael G. Newman, D.D.S.

No longer a simple choice   Until the 1970s, dental infections were analyzed quite simply: they were either sterile or bacterial (infected). If bacterial, they were assumed to be caused by either *Streptococcus* or *Staphylococcus*. With this perspective of orofacial microbiology it was no wonder that selecting an antibiotic was a simple matter. Penicillin and erythromycin were the drugs of choice, in standard doses of 250 mg qid. Little emphasis was given to the size or metabolic limitations of the patient when determining this dosage or to the predominance of anaerobes inhabiting the oral cavity.

Matching pharmacology with microbiology   **The organisms that cause orofacial infections respond to about half of the approximately 20 distinct antibiotics.** (Although a comprehensive list of proprietary drugs will contain a bewildering array of

Table 5.1   Types of bacteria in dental infections

Source of specimen	Total cases	with anaerobes	with anaerobes exclusively	with facultatives exclusively
		Number of cases		
Bacteremia secondary to tooth extraction[1]	25	21 (84%)	6 (24%)	2 (8%)
Root canal systems of necrotic teeth[2]	19	18 (95%)	13 (67%)	2 (10%)
Root canal systems of necrotic teeth[3]	55	55 (100%)	18 (33%)	0
Orofacial odontogenic infections[4]	31	29 (95%)	13 (42%)	Unable to determine
Periodontal abscess[5]	9	9 (100%)	0	0
Abscessed teeth in children[6]	12	12 (100%)	8 (67%)	0
Dental abscesses of endodontic origin[7]	10	9 (90%)	6 (60%)	1 (10%)

hundreds of antibiotic agents, most are close chemical analogs or the same agents marketed under different brand names.) Most dental infections are caused by mixtures of facultative and anaerobic bacteria, but the anaerobic bacteria usually dominate[1-12] (see **Table 5.1**). From 85% to 100% of orofacial infections involve anaerobes; 30% to 60% of these infections involve anaerobes exclusively. Facultative bacteria in orofacial infections are seldom present alone. **Tables 1.1** to **1.3** (see chapter 1) and many chapters in this book detail the microbiota of specific orofacial infections. The antibiotics with pharmacologies suited to combat infections of this microbiological nature are examined in the next pages. **Table 5.2** gives pharmacokinetic data for the most common antibiotics.

The penicillins

The penicillins are a group of natural (from *Penicillium notatum*) and synthetic compounds with different properties of antibacterial action and similar propensities for allergenicity. They have low toxicity to the host, potent antibacterial action on susceptible species, and allergic cross-reactivity with each other.

Of the 3,000 or so penicillins developed, the derivatives discussed below are useful in dental practice. All these compounds share a common structural property. They are β-lactams and they have the β-lactamic chain incorporated in the β-lactamic ring.

All these compounds act on the development (formation) of the bacterial cell wall. The β-lactamic area of the antibiotic is structurally similar to part of the muramic acid pentapeptide, a fundamental component of the bacterial cell wall. Thus, these antibiotics interfere with bacterial cell wall synthesis and development, leading to cell lysis. The main bacterial defense against these compounds is the production of enzymes — β-lactamases (see chapter 3) — that open the lactamic ring and destroy its activity.

Penicillin G (benzyl penicillin)

Absorption   Oral absorption is erratic. Parenteral route is preferred to obtain complete absorption, though chances of allergy developing are increased by injection.

Distribution   Widely distributed throughout the body. The half-life in serum is short (approximately 20 minutes), and in order to maintain adequate serum levels, continued administration of high dosages is necessary.

Excretion   Cleared by renal system. Dosage in patients with impaired renal function should be decreased. In order to prolong the effect of this drug, different formulations have been developed. **Penicillin procaine** can be administered intramuscularly and is dissolved slowly; 4 million units (4 mg) can inhibit sensitive pathogens during 36 hours. **Penicillin benzathine** is even less soluble, and adequate serum concentrations can be demonstrated during several weeks.

Table 5.2 Pharmacokinetics of common antibiotics

Drug	Route	Primary excretion route	Percent serum protein binding	Duration	Removed by	
					Hemodialysis	Peritoneal dialysis
Penicillins						
Ampicillin	Oral/IM/IV	Renal	20	500 mg dose peaks at 4 μg/mL at 1h; 1.5h half-life	Yes	No
Amoxicillin	Oral/IM/IV	Renal	20	500 mg dose peaks at 2h; 1.5h half-life at 7 μg/mL	Yes	No
Augmentin	Oral/IM/IV	Renal	20	500 mg dose peaks at 2h; 1.5h half-life at 7 μg/mL	Yes	No
Bacampicillin	Oral	Renal	20	800 mg dose peaks at 12–14 μg/mL at 1h; 1h half-life	Yes	No
Penicillin G	Oral	Renal	60	Peaks in 45 min	Yes	No
Aqueous	IM	Renal	60	Peak serum level 8 μg/mL; unchanged in urine; 2h half-life	Yes	No
Procaine	IM	Renal	60	Peaks at 1 μg/mL; 60%–90% excreted in first hour	Yes	No
Penicillin V	Oral	Renal	80	Peaks at 6 μg/mL at 45 min; 1h half-life	Yes	No
Penicillinase-Resistant Penicillin						
Methicillin	IM/IV	Renal	40	Peak serum level at 45 min; 1h half-life	No	No
Nafcillin	Oral/IM/IV	Renal	90	Peak level in 1.5h; 45 min half-life	No	No
Oxacillin	Oral/IM/IV	Renal	90	Peak level in 30 min; 45 min half-life	No	No

Cloxacillin	Oral	Renal	93–95	Peak level in 1.5h; peak serum level at 10 µg/mL; 45 min half-life	No	No
Dicloxacillin	Oral	Renal	96	Peak level at 45 min; 45 min half-life	No	No
Cephalosporins						
Cephalexin	Oral	Renal	5–15	Peak serum level 17 µg/mL; rapidly absorbed; eliminated from blood within 8h; 40 min half-life; about 60% excreted unchanged in urine within 2h	Yes	Yes
Tetracyclines						
Tetracycline HCl	Oral	1° Renal/2° Biliary	20–25	Peak serum level 3 µg/mL; 60% excreted unchanged in urine; 6–10h half-life	Yes	Yes
Minocycline	Oral	1° Biliary/2° Renal	75	Peak serum level 0.7–4.5 µg/mL; 5%–10% excreted in urine unchanged; 11–20h half-life	Yes	No
Doxycycline	Oral	1° Biliary/2° Renal	90	Peak serum level 1–6 µg/mL; 12–22h half-life	No	No
Erythromycins						
Erythromycin (base)	Oral	1° Hepatic/2° Renal	70	Peak serum level 1 µg/mL; 1.5h half-life	No	No
Erythromycin ethylsuccinate	Oral	Hepatic		Peak serum level 1 µg/mL; 1.5h half-life	No	No
Clindamycin	Oral	Hepatic	Very high	Peak level 45 min at 5 µg/mL; absorption rapid—not dependent on food; 2h half-life	No	No
Metronidazole	Oral	Renal	<20	12 µg/mL serum level at 500 mg dose; 8h half-life	No	No

Mode of action   Inhibits cell wall synthesis, leading to loss of cell wall integrity.

Adverse effects   The penicillins are probably the least toxic antibiotics in use; however, the prevalence of indirect toxicity (hypersensitivity) is increasing. The following are some adverse effects:

1. Fatal anaphylaxis, estimated to occur in one in 10,000 users.
2. Diarrhea, which in many cases may be minimized by taking the penicillin dose with two or three tablespoons of yogurt or the equivalent of acidophilus milk or a lactobacillum tablet.
3. At high dose it can have a toxic effect that can cause hemolytic anemias of an immunologic type, encephalitis, and nephritis.

General indications   Mild to moderately severe infections that are susceptible to relatively low tissue levels of penicillin. Many *Actinobacillus* strains are resistant (see chapter 11). They possess a spectrum that includes the majority of normal pathogenic bacteria; however, their clinical utility has diminished because currently many organisms produce β-lactamase.

Spectrum

1. Anaerobic gram-positive organisms such as: *Actinomyces, Bifidobacterium, Eubacterium, Peptococcus*, and *Peptostreptococcus*
2. Anaerobic gram-negative organisms such as: **some** *Bacteroides, Fusobacterium*, and *Veillonella*; rarely *Bacteroides fragilis*
3. Susceptible *Pneumococcus, Streptococcus*, some *Staphylococcus, Meningococcus*, and *Gonococcus*

Penicillin V (phenoxymethyl penicillin)

Identical to penicillin G except that penicillin V is not broken down by gastric acid and is therefore absorbed well orally (see **Fig. 5.1**).

Ampicillin

The main differences between ampicillin and its esters (bacampicillin) and ampicillin analogs (amoxicillin) are more pharmacologic than antibacterial. In general these drugs are slightly less active than benzylpenicillin against gram-positive cocci but are more active against gram-negative cocci and bacilli. They are sensitive to β-lactamases.

Ampicillin is very similar to penicillin but is effective against a slightly broader range of organisms, including *Proteus* sp. and *Haemophilus influenzae*, which may be found in sinus infections of dental origin and in medically compromised patients. The concurrent administration of **allopurinol** and ampicillin tends to increase the incidence of rashes as compared with patients who receive ampicillin alone. The oral absorption

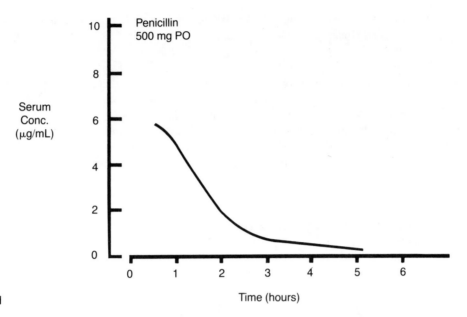

Fig. 5.1

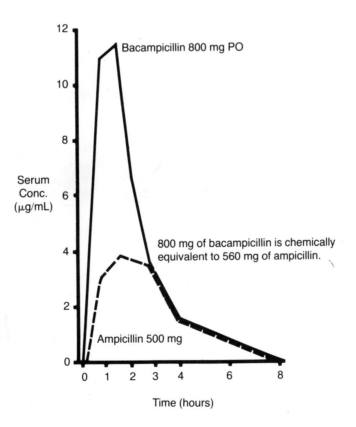

Fig. 5.2

of ampicillin is low; only 20% to 40% of the drug is eliminated by urine. Amoxicillin has approximately double the absorption of ampicillin, and its bactericidal action is quicker.

Bacampicillin (Spectrobid®)   The ethoxycarbonyloxyethel ester of ampicillin. When taken orally, it provides plasma levels equal to those obtained by IV ampicillin or amoxicillin at equivalent doses (see **Fig. 5.2**). This drug can be dosed twice a day, which can result in better patient compliance than a drug requiring more frequent dosing. Any organism sensitive to penicillin will usually be sensitive to ampicillin or bacampicillin. **Bacampicillin should *not* be coadministered with Antabuse (disulfiram).** This will produce vomiting.

Penicillinase-resistant penicillins

This group of semisynthetic penicillin agents consists of **methicillin, cloxacillin**, and **dicloxacillin**. They are resistant to penicillinase (β-lactamase) and are indicated for infections known by culture identification (see chapter 3) to be caused by penicillinase secreting *Staphylococcus*. They are also shown by antibiotic susceptibility testing to be susceptible to semisynthetic penicillins.

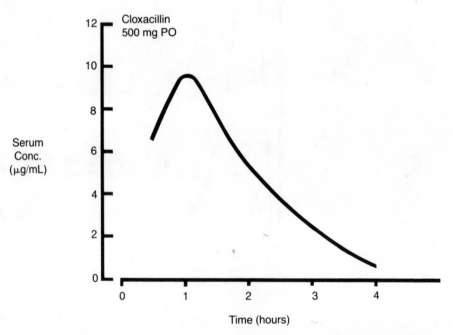

Serum Conc. (μg/mL)

Cloxacillin 500 mg PO

Time (hours)

Fig. 5.3

Methicillin (dimethyloxyphenyl penicillin) Because this drug is deactivated by gastric acids, it must be injected to be effective. Primarily for hospital use.

Cloxacillin and dicloxacillin Both of these agents are well-absorbed orally because they are gastric-acid stable. They are also β-lactamase resistant (see **Fig. 5.3**).

Inhibitors of β-lactamase These agents are β-lactams lacking antibacterial action. When associated with a drug like amoxicillin they protect this drug against lactamase-hydrolysis. Clavulanic acid, associated with amoxicillin, is the best known of these inhibitors. It is incorporated into the drug **Augmentin®**. It increases the spectrum of activity of the amoxicillin, including all bacteria capable of synthesizing β-lactamase.

Recommendation summary: The penicillins

A penicillin remains the first drug of choice for anaerobic infections above the diaphragm — including odontogenic infections.[3,4,6,8-11] A penicillinase-resistant penicillin should only be prescribed when the predominant infecting organisms have been identified as penicillinase-producing, commonly *Staphylococcus*. However, because of the increasing numbers of bacteria capable of penicillinase synthesis, the use of combinations of ampicillin or amoxicillin with β-lactamase inhibitors will increase in the future.

The nonpenicillins

Cephalexin

Description A derivative of 7-aminocephalosporinic acid, which was originally derived from a Sardinian fungus. A member of the group cephalosporins, which are β-lactams but are less susceptible than penicillins to β-lactamase action.

Absorption Adequate absorption is obtained following oral administration.

Distribution Bound to plasma proteins.

Excretion Cleared by renal glomerular filtration.

Mode of action Inhibits bacterial cell wall synthesis.

Adverse effects Nephrotoxicity has been reported as well as cross allergenicity with penicillin-allergic patients. Therefore, **great caution should be exercised when**

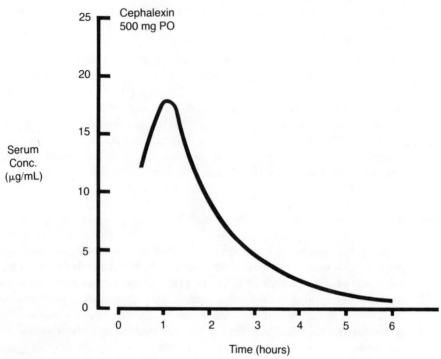

Fig. 5.4

considering this drug for a penicillin-allergic patient. Its spectrum is broader than penicillins because it includes most gram-negative cocci and bacilli.

Spectrum Infections caused by β-hemolytic *Streptococcus, Staphylococcus, Streptococcus pneumonia, Escherichia coli, Proteus mirabilis, Klebsiella, H. influenzae*, and *Neisseria*.

Recommendation Cephalexin is *not* the first drug of choice for most types of dental infections.[12,13] It does not provide an advantage over the use of benzylpenicillin or the aminopenicillins (ampicillin or amoxicillin). Although broad in its spectrum, it does not coincide with the *predominant* bacteria isolated from most odontogenic infections (see **Fig. 5.4**). This drug should be reserved for life-threatening infections and for hospital use. It should be used only if antibiotic susceptibility tests indicate it is the most efficacious drug for the individual.

Clindamycin

Description A chemical derivative of lincomycin produced by *Streptomyces lincolnensis*. Clindamycin is active against most anaerobic bacteria, and some authors consider it the drug of choice against infections caused by anaerobic bacteria resistant to penicillins.

Absorption Almost total, after oral administration.

Distribution Passes readily into most tissues. A special and important property of this drug is its active transport to the interior of macrophages and polymorphonuclear leukocytes, which explains the high concentration of this drug in abscesses.

Excretion Metabolized in liver and excreted in bile. Dosage should be decreased if the patient has impaired hepatic function.

Mode of action Binds to 50S ribosomes, leading to inhibition of protein synthesis.

Adverse effects The most frequent adverse reaction is diarrhea, which occurs in 10% to 20% of individuals. It is probably a consequence of direct action of this drug on the intestinal mucosae and microbiota. The most important gastrointestinal complication is psuedomembranous colitis (PMC) induced by *Clostridium difficile*. This organism is more resistant to clindamycin and survives antibiotic therapy. In nondental and dental infections (this disease process has also been reported in the absence of antibiotic therapy and in patients receiving ampicillin, cephalosporins, erythromycin, penicillin, and tetracycline) it is treated by oral vancomycin. Another frequent side effect is the appearance of a *morbiliform eruption* (3% to 5% of individuals).

Indications and spectrum For *serious* infections caused by aerobic gram-positive cocci, including *Staphylococcus* and *Pneumococcus*. Further indications are for serious infections caused by anaerobic gram-negative rods such as *Bacteroides* (especially *B. fragilis*) and *Fusobacterium*; anaerobic gram-positive rods such as *Actinomyces, Eubacterium*, and *Propionibacterium*; anaerobic gram-positive cocci such as *Peptococcus* and *Peptostreptococcus*; and anaerobic gram-negative cocci such as *Veillonella*. *This agent should be considered only with medical consultation in penicillin-allergic patients when serious anaerobic infection is present.*

Discussion Clindamycin produces excellent results against most anaerobic organisms, including those found in oral and odontogenic infections. Kannangara et al.[11] reported a high cure rate for patients with dental infections either by using clindamycin initially or by changing to clindamycin following failure with conventional penicillin therapy. Oral administration of clindamycin at a dose of 300 mg will produce peak serum levels of 3 to 5 mg/mL. This compares favorably to the average minimum inhibitory concentration (MIC) for *B. fragilis*, which is 2 μg/mL.

The most significant adverse reaction that has been associated with clindamycin, as well as other antibiotics, has been the finding of pseudomembranous colitis. This problem has been reported in nondental patients, secondary to ampicillin,[14] cephalosporins such as cephalexin,[15] erythromycin,[16] penicillin,[17] and tetracycline.[18] A number of current papers report PMC in the absence of antibiotic therapy.[19-23] The first reported case of pseudomembranous colitis, in 1893, preceded the antibiotic era by some 40

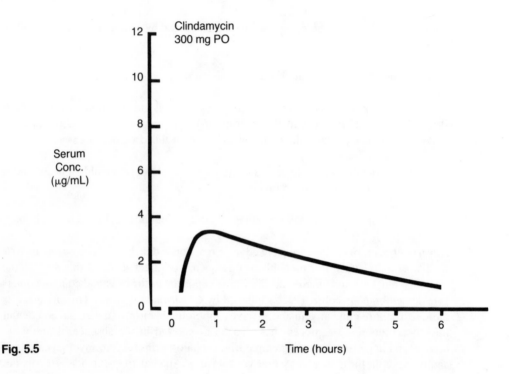

Fig. 5.5

years.[24] The precise etiology of pseudomembranous colitis has been shown to be an overgrowth of *C. difficile*, which explains why this disease process can occur in the absence of antibiotic therapy (see **Fig. 5.5**).

Recommendation   Clindamycin is most likely to be used by a specialist for *serious* infections of known etiology that have failed to respond to a first-choice antibiotic, usually a penicillin. It can also be used as first-line drug for the penicillin-allergic patient who presents with a *serious* infection, or for the medically compromised patient.[3,6,10,11,15,25] Because serious diarrhea can be a side effect, **consultation with the patient's physician is indicated.**

Erythromycin

Description   Produced by *Streptomyces erytheus* in the year 1952. Erythromycins are classified as macrolide antibiotics. They are one of the safer antibiotics in use and they are often a satisfactory alternative to penicillin, particularly in patients allergic to penicillin. It is available for oral administration in four forms: *(1)* erythromycin base; *(2)* as a salt, erythromycin stearate; *(3)* as an ester, erythromycin ethylsuccinate; and *(4)* as erythromycin estolate, a salt of the ester.

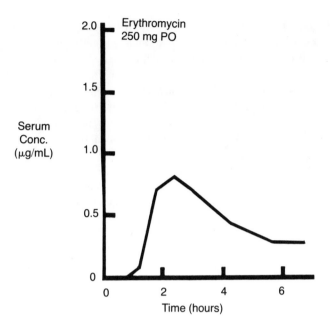

Fig. 5.6

Absorption Erythromycin base is destroyed by gastric acid, so it should be administered in an enteric-coated tablet that is resistant to acids (E-mycin®) or capsules containing enteric-coated pellets (ERYC®). Erythromycin stearate and estolate are less sensitive to gastric acid.

Distribution To most body tissues, with peak blood levels 1 to 4 hours after ingestion. The serum concentrations obtained with the base or with stearate are similar; however, *with the estolate they are three to four times higher* (see "Adverse effects," below).

Excretion Via urine and bile.

Mode of action Binds to the 50S ribosomes, thereby inhibiting protein synthesis.

Adverse effects Cholestatic jaundice associated with the estolate (Ilosone®) form, and theophylline toxicity in patients concurrently taking erythromycin. Gastrointestinal symptoms (vomiting, nausea, and diarrhea) are very common.

Indications and spectrum Erythromycin is the drug of choice for diphtheria, Legionnaires' disease, and pertussis.[26] Further indications include *Mycoplasma pneumonia*, streptococcal and staphylococcal infections, tetanus, syphilis, and gonorrhea.[27] It is not the drug of choice for typical anaerobic dental infections.

79

Discussion   The erythromycins are not particularly effective against obligate anaerobic organisms at levels that can be obtained orally, although they can be effective if infused intravenously to achieve high enough serum levels.[9,28,29] When it was thought that *Staphylococcus* and *Streptococcus* were the predominant bacteria in odontogenic infections, there was merit to considering erythromycin as an alternative to penicillin. Reports appear in the literature from time to time suggesting that, based on clinical observation, erythromycin is efficacious for most dental infections. Success was probably due to adequate debridement, removal of necrotic substrate, and drainage.

Recommendation   Erythromycin can be used for the penicillin-allergic patient who presents with a nonserious infection. For the penicillin-allergic patient who does not respond to erythromycin for a nonserious infection, a tetracycline such as doxycycline or minocycline is suggested[3,10,25] (see **Fig. 5.6**).

Tetracyclines

Description   A group of similar natural (from the *Streptomyces* sp.) and synthetic compounds with similar properties.

Absorption   Tetracycline hydrochloride is approximately 70% absorbed orally. Antacids and dairy products will inhibit absorption because tetracycline binds to calcium. Doxycycline (Vibramycin®) and minocycline (Minocin®) are approximately 100% and 95% absorbed, respectively. Doxycycline may be taken with food or milk.

Distribution   Wide. Concentrates in gingival fluid at higher concentrations than in plasma; this is important for periodontal infections (see chapter 11).

Excretion   Via renal system by glomerular filtration. It is accumulated in case of renal insufficiency.

Mode of action   Binds to the 30S ribosomes, leading to inhibition of protein synthesis. It is a bacteriostatic agent.

Adverse effects   Superinfection (see chapter 10), diarrhea, and staining of calcified tissues. Staining of teeth in children less than 12 years old. For this reason tetracyclines should not be used with pregnant women after the fifth month of pregnancy (see chapter 19). May inactivate contraceptives. Photosensitivity reactions are common to any of the tetracyclines. Hepatotoxicity and nephrotoxicity can be caused at high doses. Vestibular alterations (vertigo, tinnitus) are common with the use of minocycline.

Spectrum   Infections caused by *Actinomyces, Actinobacillus, Bacteroides* sp., *Propionibacterium, Clostridium, Eubacterium, Peptococcus*, some *B. fragilis*, and *Fusobacterium*.

Discussion   Tetracyclines are effective against many species of obligate anaerobic

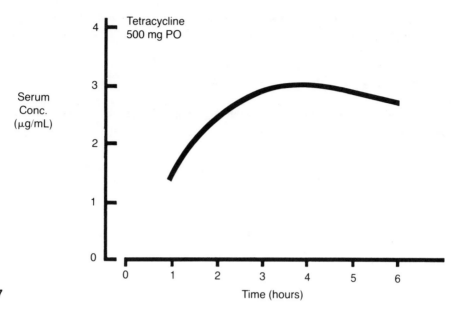

Fig. 5.7

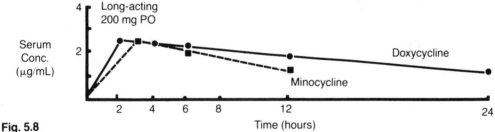

Fig. 5.8

organisms, but their efficacy has been hampered because some strains of bacteria have developed resistance. Tetracyclines have been used successfully in an adjunctive treatment mode for patients with localized juvenile periodontitis (see chapter 19).

Because tetracyclines are purported to result in frequent fungal overgrowth in mucous membranes of the gastrointestinal tract and vagina, mixtures of tetracyclines and antifungal agents are available. Although such mixtures may have some rational basis in patients who are diabetic, debilitated, or receiving adrenal corticosteroids, there is no convincing evidence in the medical-dental literature that the mixtures result in decreased fungal infections in these patients.

Recommendation **Doxycycline** (Vibramycin) and **minocycline** (Minocin) are the best-absorbed tetracyclines and can be dosed once or twice a day, which may enhance patient compliance. Tetracyclines are preferred over erythromycin for the penicillin-allergic patient who presents with a nonserious infection caused by any of the organisms listed above (see **Figs. 5.7** and **5.8**).

Metronidazole

Description   A nonnaturally occurring compound derived from nitroimidazole.

Absorption   Well-absorbed orally.

Distribution   Passes readily into most tissues and into saliva.

Excretion   Via renal system.

Mode of action   Reduction of nitro group, which in turn disrupts DNA synthesis, leading to cell death.

Adverse effects   Toxic reactions with disulfiram. Possible Antabuse® effect with alcohol. Potentiates the effects of anticoagulants. Metallic taste, nausea, large doses may cause peripheral neuropathy.

Indications   Should be considered for the penicillin-allergic patient for serious anaerobic infections. It is active against practically all gram-negative anaerobic rods and clostridium. The aerobic and microaerophilic bacteria are usually resistant.

Spectrum   Infections involving *Bacteroides* sp., including the *fragilis* group (*fragilis, distasonis, ovatus, thetaiotaomicron, vulgatus, gingivalis*), *Fusobacterium, Clostridium, Eubacterium, Peptococcus*, and *Peptostreptococcus*.

Recommendation   For the patient who presents with a serious infection of dental origin and is allergic to penicillin or has failed with penicillin therapy (see **Fig. 5.9**). Because 85% of dental infections involve obligate anaerobes (see **Table 5.1**), its rationale for use in dental infections is well founded. It is recommended for infections of dental or periodontal origin in individuals allergic to penicillin. In some specific instances, such as ANUG or very advanced or refractory periodontitis, its use can be considered if antimicrobial susceptibility testing indicates susceptible strains are present.

Antifungal drugs

Nystatin

Description   Obtained from *Streptomyces noursei*. Topical.

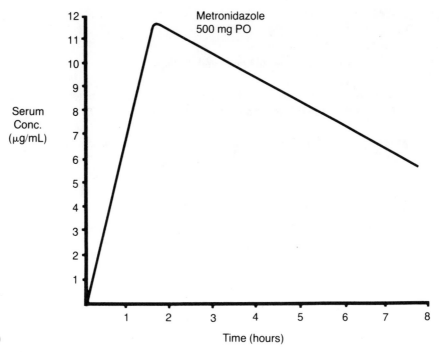

Fig. 5.9

Absorption Negligible from the intestinal tract, and not at all from skin or mucous membranes.

Mode of action Binds to ergosterol within the membranes of sensitive fungi.

Adverse effects If ingested can cause nausea, vomiting, and diarrhea.

Indications *Candida albicans* infections (candidiasis).

Discussion Candidiasis in the oral cavity can result when the balance of the microbial flora changes because of antibiotic therapy or severe illness (see chapter 10). In the resulting disease, known as candidiasis or thrush, the oral mucosa is inflamed and painful and covered with a white membrane. If antibiotic therapy precipitated the infection, the antibiotic therapy should be discontinued if possible.

Recommendation Treatment with nystatin will usually be effective. However, for deep-seated fungal infections, **amphotericin B** may be prescribed under the direction of a medical specialist.

Ketoconazol

Description   Ketoconazol (Nizoral®) is an antifungal drug for oral treatment of systemic fungal infections and oral candidiasis.

Absorption   Its absorption from the gastrointestinal tract is better than that of nystatin. It is metabolized in the liver and only small amounts are found in urine and feces.

Mode of action   Ketoconazol interferes with fungus plasma membrane synthesis, leading to membrane disorganization and cell lysis.

Adverse effects   The most common are nausea and pruritus. Less frequently, gastrointestinal problems, nervousness, and liver dysfunction.

Indications   Mainly for oral candidiasis in patients resistant to nystatin as well as for therapy of systemic fungal infections in immunocompromised patients. It is very commonly used in HIV-oral fungal infections. For deep-seated or systemic fungal infections that are nonresponsive to both nystatin and ketoconazol, parenteral administration of **amphotericin B** is considered to be the treatment of choice, but it should be prescribed under the direction of a medical specialist.

Myconazole (Monistat) is not intended for topical oral use. However, ketoconazole, taken as a once daily tablet (Nizoral) for 7 to 14 days, appears to supplement topical Clotrimazole (Mycelex) for treatment of oral candidiasis. Fluconazole is also a promising agent for treatment of this clinical condition (see chapter 8).

Antiviral agents

Description   These agents produce their effect by stimulating the host to form antibodies against infected cells, by nonspecific resistance, by interference with infected cell activity, or by diminishing the symptomatology. The different antiviral agents are active selectively against either RNA or DNA virus.

Idoxuridine   A synthetic analog of pyrimidine; inhibits the enzymes of the DNA pathway and competes with timidine in the incorporation of viral and cellular DNA. It is only prepared for ophthalmic use in the treatment of herpes simplex keratitis. Today it is not an antiviral agent of first choice for human herpes infections because of its high toxicity.

Vidarabine   Belongs to a series of compounds used in cancer therapy. It also interferes with DNA synthesis. It is used for herpes keratitis in a topical preparation and via parenteral use for herpes simplex encephalitis.

Acyclovir   An acyclic nucleoside analogous to purine. Its antiviral activity depends on its intracellular conversion into a triphosphate derivative that inhibits DNA-polymerase. It is a very specific and potent DNA-antiviral agent because it binds 100%

better to viral timidin kinase than to cellular kinase, and it is phosphorylated by the cellular enzyme much quicker than by the cellular enzyme.

Both type 1 and 2 herpes simplex virus and varicella-zoster virus are highly susceptible to this drug. Epstein-Barr virus has an intermediate susceptibility, and cytomegalovirus is usually resistant. It has been used with success in recurrent orofacial herpes simplex infections, recurrent herpes genitalis, and in the management of herpes labialis. The viruses can become resistant to this drug by mutation, precluding indiscriminate use of these agents. Acyclovir should only be used in highly susceptible individuals and immunocompromised patients.

Administration can be oral, topical, ointment, and parenteral. Adverse reactions are more common with intravenous use and are mainly nausea and vomiting as well as neurologic and liver reactions. The incidence of adverse effects with oral administration is much lower. With ointment application there is usually a transient pain or burning sensation at the application site, but topical treatment is well tolerated overall.

Other antiviral agents such as **Bromovinil-2′-desoxiuridine** (BVDU), **citarabine, 6-azauridine, fluoriodine-aracitosine** (FIAC), and **Fosfonoformate** have also been used as anti-DNA viruses but not in the treatment of orofacial viral infections.

Summary of recommendations

If an antibiotic is necessary, an agent with a spectrum that coincides with the anticipated microbiology at the site of the infection should be selected, and a dosage that will produce an adequate serum/tissue level should be prescribed (see **Tables 5.3** and **5.4** for dosage guidelines). Collection of a culture specimen is recommended for establishing a microbiological diagnosis that can be used if the patient fails to respond to an agent or dosage chosen on empirical evidence (see chapter 4).

Which drug to use

1. A penicillin derivative such as **ampicillin, amoxicillin**, or **Augmentin** is recommended for the nonpenicillin-allergic patient who presents with a serious infection, provided adequate laboratory support for culture and susceptibility testing is readily available.[30–33]
2. An ampicillin such as **bacampicillin** should be considered if the infection involves the sinus.
3. **Metronidazole** or **clindamycin** is recommended for beginning treatment of a serious infection in the patient who is penicillin-allergic, medically compromised, or failing to respond to penicillin therapy.
4. **Penicillin derivatives, tetracycline**, or **metronidazole** are preferred over erythromycin for the patient who presents with a nonserious infection.
5. Some infections may require specific antibiotics, e.g., tetracycline for localized juvenile periodontitis.

Table 5.3   Average oral doses recommended for adults
Assumes 150-pound patient with normal renal and hepatic functions.
Actual doses vary with severity of infection.

Antibiotic	Usual dose
Penicillins	
Ampicillin	250–500 mg q6h
Amoxicillin	250–500 mg q6h
Augmentin	250–500 mg q6h
Bacampicillin	400–800 mg q12h
Penicillin G	400,000–600,000 units q6h
Penicillin V	500 mg q6h
Oxacillin	500 mg q6h
Nafcillin	250 mg–1 gr q4–6h
Cloxacillin	500 mg q6h
Dicloxacillin	500 mg q6h
Cephalosporins	
Cephalexin	250–500 mg q6h
Cefaclor	250 mg q6h
Cephadrine	500 mg q6h
Tetracyclines	
Tetracycline HCl	250 mg q6h
Doxycycline	200 mg initially, then 100 mg q12h
Minocycline	200 mg initially, then 100 mg q12h
Erythromycins	
Erythromycin base	250–500 mg q6h
Erythromycin ethylsuccinate	400 mg q6h
Clindamycin	300 mg initially, then 150 mg q8h
Metronidazole	250 mg q8h

What the patient needs to know

As with all medications, the patient must be told of:

1. The benefits to be gained by taking the drug
2. Possible side effects
3. Potential outcome if medication is not taken at all or is not taken as directed

Table 5.4 Average doses recommended for children

Actual doses are based on infection severity, child's age, and renal and hepatic clearances. ·

Antibiotic	Usual dose*
Ampicillin	50 mg/kg/d (For severe infections the drug should be administered parenterally.)
Cephalexin	25–50 mg/kg in divided doses (In severe infections the dose can be doubled.)
Clindamycin, oral†	15–25 mg/kg/d in 3–4 doses; more severe infections, 25–40 mg/kg/d in 3–4 doses, with medical consultation
Erythromycin (base)‡	30–50 mg/kg/d in divided doses (Doses can be doubled in more severe infections.)

Erythromycin ethylsuccinate‡	Body weight	Daily dose
	Less than 10 lb	30–50 mg/kg/d
		15–25 mg/lb/d
	10–15 lb	200 mg
	16–25 lb	400 mg
	25–50 lb	800 mg
	51–100 lb	1,200 mg
	More than 100 lb	1,600 mg

Penicillin G, oral; and Penicillin V	15–50 mg (25,000–90,000 units)/kg/d in 3–6 divided doses
Tetracycline HCl	More than 8 years of age: 25–50 mg/kg or 10–20 mg/lb, divided into 4 doses

*kg refers to child's weight.
†Taken with a full glass of water.
‡Taken before meals.

References

1. Crawford, J.J., et al. 1974. Bacteremia after tooth extraction studied with the aid of prereduced anaerobically sterilized culture media. *Appl. Microbiol.* 27:927–932.

2. Sundqvist, G.K. 1976. Bacteriologic studies of necrotic dental pulps. Odontological Dissertation No. 7, University of Umea, Umea, Sweden.

3. Goodman, A.D. 1977. Isolation of anaerobic bacteria from the root canal systems of necrotic teeth by use of a transport solution. *Oral Surg.* 43:766–770.

4. Chow, A.W., Roser, S.M., and Brady, F.A. 1978. Orofacial odontogenic infections. *Ann. Intern. Med.* 88:392–402.

5. Newman, M.G., and Sims, T.N. 1979. The predominant cultivable microbiota of the periodontal abscess. *J. Periodontol.* 50:350–354.

6. Brook, I., Grimm, S., and Kielich, R.B. 1981. Bacteriology of acute periapical abscess in children. *J. Endodontol.* 7:378–380.

7. Williams, B.L., McCann, G.F., and Schoenknecht, F.D. 1983. Bacteriology of dental abscesses of endodontic origin. *J. Clin. Microbiol.* 18:770–774.

8. Bartlett, J.G., and O'Keefe, P. 1979. The bacteriology of perimandibular space infections. *J. Oral Surg.* 37:407–409.

9. Finegold, S.M., and George, L.W. 1989. *Anaerobic Infections in Humans.* New York: Academic Press.

10. Goodman, A.D. 1982. Current microbiology, laboratory procedures, and antimicrobial considerations for odontogenic infections. *Boston Univ. Endodont. J.* 7:10–11.

11. Kannangara, D.W., Thadepalli, H., and McQuirtir, J.L. 1980. Bacteriology and treatment of dental infections. *Oral Surg.* 50:103–109.

12. Hook, E.W. 1977. *Current Concepts of Infectious Diseases.* New York: John Wiley & Sons.

13. AMA Drug Evaluations. 1977. 3rd ed. Littleton, Mass.: Publishing Sciences Group, Inc.

14. Finch, R.G. 1979. Relapse of pseudomembranous colitis after vancomycin therapy. *Lancet* 17 Nov. 1979: 1076–1077.

15. Bartlett, J.G. 1979. Cephalosporin-associated pseudomembranous colitis due to *Clostridium difficile.* *JAMA* 242:2683–2685.

16. Gantz, M.N., et al. 1979. Pseudomembranous colitis associated with erythromycin therapy. *Ann. Intern. Med.* 91:866–867.

17. deMulder, P. 1978. Penicillin associated colitis. *Lancet* 12 Nov. 1978: 1151.

18. Mayer, I.E., et al. 1979. Fecal *Clostridia* species in patients with pseudomembranous colitis and inflammatory bowel disease. *Am. J. Gastroenterol.* 72:339.

19. Scopes, J.W. 1980. Pseudomembranous colitis and sudden infant death. The Lancet 24 May 1980: 1144.

20. Peiken, S.R. 1980. Role of *Clostridium difficile* in a case of non-antibiotic associated pseudomembranous colitis. *Gastroentology* 79:948–951.

21. Wald, A. 1980. Non-associated pseudomembranous colitis due to toxin producing *Clostridia.* *Ann. Intern. Med.* 92:798–799.

22. Howard, J.M. 1980. Spontaneous pseudomembranous colitis. *Br. Med. J.* 2 Aug. 1980:356.

23. Moskovitz, M. 1981. Recurrent pseudomembranous colitis unassociated with prior antibiotic therapy. *Arch. Intern. Med.* 141:663–671.

24. Finney, J.M.T. 1893. Gastroenterostomy for cicatrizing ulcer of the pylorus. *Bull. Johns Hopkins Hosp.* 4:53.

25. Aderhold, L. 1981. Bacteriology of dentogenous pyogenic infections. *Oral Surg.* 52:587.

26. Mandell, G.L., and Sande, M.A. 1980. Antimicrobial agents: general considerations. pp. 1138–1140. *In* A.G. Gilman et al. (eds.) *Goodman and Gilman's The Pharmacological Basis of Therapeutics.* 6th ed. New York: Macmillan Publishing Co.

27. Sande, M.A., and Mandell, G.L. 1980. Antimicrobial agents: general considerations. pp. 1085, 1182, 1225. *In* A.G. Gilman et al. (eds.) *Goodman and Gilman's The Pharmacological Basis of Therapeutics.* 6th ed. New York: Macmillan Publishing Co.

28. Martin, W.J. 1972. In vitro antimicrobial susceptibility of anaerobic bacteria isolated from clinical specimens. *Antimicrob. Agents Chemother.* 1:148.

29. Sapico, F.L. 1972. Standardized disc susceptibility testing of anaerobic bacteria. *Antimicrob. Agents Chemother.* 2:320.

30. Wise, R. 1982. Penicillins and cephalosporins: Antimicrobial and pharmacological properties. *Lancet* 2:140–143.

31. Kucers, A. 1982. Cloramphenicol, erythromycin, vancomycin and tetracyclines. *Lancet* 2:425–429.

32. Bartlett, J.G. 1982. Antianaerobic antimicrobial agents. *Lancet* 2:478–481.

33. Wust, J., and Wilkius, T.D. 1978. Effect of clavulanic acid on anaerobic bacteria resistant to β-lactam antibiotics. *Antimicrob. Agents Chemother.* 13:130–133.

CHAPTER 6

Topical Antimicrobial Agents: General Principles and Delivery Systems

Kenneth S. Kornman, D.D.S., Ph.D.

Delivery of antibacterial agents to the oral cavity may involve three approaches: *(1)* systemic, *(2)* topical application, and *(3)* controlled release. The relative merits and limitations of the three techniques have been extensively reviewed for medicine and dentistry.[1-3] In dentistry, topical agents may be applied professionally, as with some topical fluorides, or by the patient. This chapter will emphasize what will be referred to as *patient-applied local delivery* and will include topical application of agents by means of oral rinsing or irrigation. *"Controlled-release" delivery* of drugs may involve the implantation of minipumps to deliver agents systemically on a regular schedule, as with insulin pumps for diabetics. In dentistry, however, controlled-release delivery generally involves topical application of drugs, and the term will be used in that manner. Topical antimicrobials, as currently used in dentistry, may therefore be applied by patient-applied local delivery or controlled-release delivery.

Historical perspective　The earliest antimicrobial agents were topical. They were naturally occurring antiseptics (i.e., chemical compounds that kill microbes on exposed surfaces). Topical antimicrobials work by denaturing proteins, disrupting cell membranes, or interfering with enzyme activity. They alter the structure and function not only of microorganisms but of mammalian cells. This lack of specificity and substantial tissue toxicity presented major problems for the use of early topical antimicrobials.

　With the development of systemic antibiotics, the issues of specificity and toxicity at first appeared to have been resolved. It was only natural to try the new systemic agents as locally applied topical antimicrobials. The early experiences with topical antibiotics and an increased understanding of immunology led to the recognition that allergic hypersensitivity reactions were increased when antibiotics were used topically. This observation, plus the explosive development of new antibiotics during the 1960s and 1970s, produced a general concept that topical antibiotics, and by association topical antimicrobials, were undesirable, less-advanced approaches to therapy.

Table 6.1 Patient-applied local delivery of antibacterial therapy

Advantages	Disadvantages
• No gastric upset	• Difficulty retaining therapeutic levels at site—agent is easily dissolved, diluted, or washed away by saliva
• No alteration of the protective normal flora present at sites distant from the affected area	• Risk of allergy or sensitivity in host reactions
• Should not encourage the transfer of multiple antibiotic resistance between intestinal bacteria	• Produces pulses and large fluctuations in concentration
• Allows concentrated delivery of agents to the affected site without dilution throughout the entire body	• Requires frequent administration
• May be self-administered by the patient	• Requires patient compliance

In the early 1970s, an increased awareness of the side effects of systemic antibiotics, such as allergies, gastrointestinal disorders, and the development of multiple antibiotic resistance, pointed to the need for caution in the use of systemic antibiotics. During this same period clinicians began to acknowledge that the primary hypersensitivity problems with topical antibiotics were caused almost exclusively by penicillin and were not a general problem. Topical agents began to reemerge as an important and effective modality of antibacterial therapy. The most extensive development in this area has involved topical agents for dermatologic use, primarily acne.

Why use topical agents? (see **Table 6.1**)

When systemic agents are taken orally or by intramuscular injections, they are introduced in pulses that produce a peak concentration that differs in time and level for each body compartment. After the drug reaches a peak blood level there will be a decrease in concentration, the kinetics of which depend on the drug metabolism and redistribution within the individual. The systemic agent is then readministered when the concentration is thought to be reduced close to the threshold for efficacy. Thus, systemic agents are introduced in pulses with large fluctuations in concentration. In order to achieve a prolonged effect with systemic agents, one must either take frequent doses (e.g., one tablet four times daily) or have an agent that remains active and is slowly removed from the body. This latter situation often produces undesirable side effects because the periodic pulses of the drug must use relatively high levels that will approach toxicity in some individuals. In addition, high total doses must be used to achieve therapeutic levels at local sites. Perhaps the greatest concern is that wide use of oral antibiotics appears to have created resistance to multiple antibacterial agents in some bacterial strains, and resistance factors may be transferred among intestinal bacteria, thereby increasing the number of resistant bacterial strains. Such multiple resistance could limit the usefulness of several important antibacterial agents and provides one of the principle advantages of local delivery of antibacterial agents.

Treatment planning with topical antimicrobial agents

In the design of topical antimicrobial therapy, the appropriate use of agents depends on the target area to be treated and the specific goals of therapy. Once these factors have been determined, combinations of available agents and delivery systems will dictate the specific therapeutic approach for each patient. This chapter will focus on general approaches to the use of topical agents and the delivery systems available for the agents; chapter 7 discusses the specific topical agents.

Target areas (see Table 6.2)

In the oral cavity there are four primary target areas for antimicrobial therapy. These are infections *(1)* within the tissues, *(2)* on the oral mucosa, *(3)* adjacent to supragingival plaque, and *(4)* in the subgingival area.

Infections within the tissues are most commonly odontogenic in origin and are discussed in chapters 12 and 13. Acute necrotizing ulcerative gingivitis is known to involve bacterial invasion of the periodontal tissues, and some progressive forms of periodontitis are now believed to have substantial numbers of bacteria within the soft tissue. These conditions may require systemic antibiotics. Topical antimicrobials are generally not appropriate for the treatment of infections within the tissue, although some tissue-penetrating agents in controlled-release devices could theoretically establish a sufficient concentration gradient to achieve effective levels within the tissues.

The oral mucosa may be treated topically for candidiasis, viral lesions, and secondary bacterial infections of mechanical or viral lesions. Antifungal and antiviral therapies are discussed in chapter 8. Systemic agents may be used with recurrent episodes of mucosal lesions, especially in patients with some underlying immunocompromise. The supragingival area may be treated for the control of dental caries and the control of gingivitis. Topical application of antimicrobials is ideally suited for this target area. There is currently no justification for the use of systemic antimicrobial agents in the treatment of caries or gingivitis.

The subgingival area may be treated for the management of periodontitis. This area may be treated with systemic agents (see chapter 11) or topical agents. **Patient-applied oral rinses do not reach the subgingival area directly.**

Table 6.2   Antimicrobial delivery systems for different areas of the oral cavity

| | Delivery system | | |
Target Area	Systemic	Patient-applied local delivery	Controlled-release
Within tissue*	X		
Superficial layers of mucosa†	X¶	X	X
Supragingival‡		X	X
Subgingival§	X	X#	X

*Odontogenic infections, some progressive forms of periodontal disease, puncture wounds.
†Aphthous ulcers, candidiasis, viral lesions, surface disinfection.
‡Caries, gingivitis.
§Periodontitis.
¶Systemic agents are often used with recurrent mucosal lesions, especially in immunocompromised patients.
#Irrigation only, *not* rinses.

Treatment goals

The decision to use a specific antibacterial to treat a dental disease is based on the treatment goal and the treatment approach that may achieve that goal for a specific patient. It may not be sufficient to identify the goal as a reduction in the rate of caries development because different methods of reduction require different agents and vastly different treatment regimens (see **Table 6.3**). For example, topical agents can alter the caries rate by *(1)* altering the resistance of the tooth, *(2)* reducing the quantity of bacterial plaque, and *(3)* inhibiting specific caries-associated microorganisms. Loesche[4] discussed the implications to treatment of viewing plaque as a nonspecific irritant, where disease is related to the quantity of plaque, or as specific irritant, where one type of plaque bacteria has a different disease potential from another.

Control of gingivitis may involve different treatment goals (see **Table 6.4**). Many studies have demonstrated that gingivitis can be effectively controlled by reducing plaque quantity on a regular and consistent basis. This goal may be achieved by regular mechanical plaque control or by the use of topical antiplaque agents. It also appears to be possible to control gingivitis by selectively altering the plaque levels of certain microorganisms or their products. Although gingivitis is universally associated with the undisturbed maturation of supragingival plaque, there appear to be specific bacteria that are essential for this maturation to develop to the point of causing gingivitis. As discussed in chapter 7 relative to specific agents, some antimicrobials, referred to as third-generation antiplaque agents, appear to have the ability to selectively alter the supragingival plaque such that it is less pathogenic. In addition, some forms of

---

Table 6.3   Treatment goals for caries reduction

Goal	Treatment approach
Alter resistance of tooth	• Systemic fluorides (water fluoridation or fluoride supplements) during tooth development • Topical fluorides
Reduce plaque quantity	• Mechanical plaque control • Topical antiplaque agents
Inhibit caries-associated microorganisms	• Elimination of reservoirs of bacteria • Topical antibacterial agents used intensively for short periods to alter the ecological positions of these bacteria and to allow fewer pathogenic organisms to capture that ecological niche

---

Table 6.4   Treatment goals for control of gingivitis

Goal	Treatment approach
Reduce plaque quantity	• Mechanical plaque control • Topical antiplaque agents —patient-applied local delivery —controlled release
Selectively alter gingivitis-associated microorganisms or their products	• Topical antimicrobial agents (third generation) • Flush out toxic products (i.e., irrigate at the gingival margin)
Selectively alter host response to bacteria	• Combine anti-inflammatory agents with antimicrobials

---

mechanical flushing of the supragingival and marginal areas appear to effectively control gingivitis without reducing plaque quantity. More recently, there has been interest in the use of anti-inflammatory agents for controlling periodontal diseases. These agents appear unable by themselves to control gingivitis. In the future such agents may hold promise in the prevention and treatment of gingivitis if combined with mechanical or chemical approaches to reduction of the microbial load.

Adult periodontitis

Control of disease progression in periodontitis requires control of the subgingival microbiota. It is now known that there are multiple types of periodontitis that involve different host responses and different subgingival periodontal pathogens. Most importantly, some forms of periodontitis have less predictable clinical responses to conventional periodontal therapy. This discussion will focus on the role of topical antimicrobials in the management of adult periodontitis (see **Table 6.5**), the disease form most commonly seen in general practice and the disease most predictably treated by conventional therapy.

The use of antimicrobial agents in the treatment of adult periodontitis is based on current concepts of the role of subgingival microorganisms in the initiation and progression of periodontal diseases and our understanding of the interface between supragingival and subgingival bacterial accumulations. In this discussion, the term *adult periodontitis* will apply to individuals over the age of 35 years who have moderate to heavy accumulations of plaque and calculus and loss of periodontal attachment and bone involving up to 50% of the root length.

The accumulation of evidence in the past 15 years implicating specific bacteria as periodontal pathogens has led to a greater appreciation of the role of bacterial control in periodontal therapy. Current therapeutic approaches are based on the general concept that periodontal diseases can be controlled by altering the subgingival bacterial populations thought to be pathogenic and by interfering with repopulation by these bacteria. The validity of this approach in gingivitis and adult periodontitis has been clearly established by extensive clinical studies. It should be emphasized that these studies establish the *principle;* however, the specific *method* of achieving bacterial control may vary depending on the individual practitioner's orientation and expertise, as well as the availability of appropriate chemotherapeutic agents. The use of topical antimicrobials in adult periodontitis may involve a variety of therapeutic goals and

Table 6.5   Treatment goals for control of adult periodontitis

Goal	Treatment approach
Control of subgingival microbiota	• Mechanical subgingival cleaning (scaling and root planing) *plus*: —patient-applied local delivery of antimicrobials via subgingival irrigation —controlled release of antimicrobials
Prevent recolonization of subgingival area or control emergence of pathogens	• Mechanical supragingival plaque control • Chemical antiplaque agents

approaches as outlined in **Table 6.5**. *One must clearly distinguish between supra-gingival and subgingival bacterial compartments* because different bacteria reside in the two locations and control of the two ecosystems requires different approaches. It is essential to successful treatment of adult periodontitis that both the supragingival and subgingival bacterial populations be targeted.

Conventional therapy

Treatment of adult periodontitis by conventional periodontal therapy involves controlling the subgingival microbiota and preventing recolonization of this area from supragingival sources or from reemergence of residual subgingival bacterial populations. Control of the subgingival microbiota may be accomplished either by mechanical approaches alone, such as scaling and root planing, or with adjunctive antimicrobial therapy. Currently there are little data to support the adjunctive use of systemic antibiotics in adult periodontitis. It is also difficult to find data that demonstrate a significant clinical advantage when adjunctive topical antimicrobials are used with scaling and root planing as compared to scaling and root planing alone. Intuitively, adjunctive antimicrobials should offer an advantage in controlling the subgingival microbiota. It may well be that our current experimental designs and/or the limitations of our clinical measurements may limit our ability to detect such advantages. With the increased availability of diagnostic tests for monitoring subgingival pathogens or markers of tissue destruction, benefits of antimicrobial use may become more evident. **Topical antimicrobials applied by means of an oral rinse are effective only against supragingival plaque and should not be used for controlling subgingival bacteria.**

Topical agents may be applied directly to the subgingival area by means of irrigating devices. Special subgingival irrigator tips and pressure-control modifications are now available for powered oral irrigators. This is an appealing therapeutic approach, even though it requires patient compliance and dexterity, and should be evaluated more extensively. Of great interest today for controlling subgingival bacteria is the use of controlled-release devices for subgingival delivery of antimicrobials. Unlike many medical conditions, the infection in periodontitis is both localized and accessible, making it an ideal candidate for local controlled release of antimicrobials. This approach is discussed below.

After controlling the subgingival microbiota in adult periodontitis, it appears to be essential to prevent recolonization of this area or to control reemergence of pathogens that may remain in the subgingival environment. If subgingival bacterial deposits are removed but supragingival plaque is not controlled, the subgingival microbiota will return to its pretreatment status within weeks. This is seen in the patient who receives appropriate professional therapy but does not maintain adequate home care. Antiplaque agents may be effective adjuncts in this situation. In particular, antibiotic use in periodontal therapy appears to be significantly more effective when combined with good supragingival plaque control.

Table 6.6   Common types of controlled-release delivery devices

---

- Reservoirs *without* rate-controlling system
  Example: hollow fibers filled with agent. Release of agent is determined simply by diffusion out
  of the reservoir.

- Reservoirs *with* rate-controlling system
  Example: microcapsules filled with agent. Rate is controlled by solid or microporous polymer
  membrane. A single dosage might contain different microcapsules with varying
  release rates.

- Monolithic systems
  Example: agent is dispersed in inert polymeric matrix. Active ingredient is released dependent
  on the concentration gradient.

- Laminated systems
  Example: multiple layers of polymers with different diffusion characteristics. Central layers may
  be the agent reservoir with surrounding layers that limit the diffusion rate.

Delivery systems

Delivery of topical antimicrobial agents to the target areas in the oral cavity includes
oral rinses, oral irrigation, and controlled-release approaches. The advantages and
disadvantages of patient-applied local delivery including both rinses and irrigation are
described in **Table 6.1**.

Oral rinses   The primary advantages of using oral rinses to deliver antimicrobial
agents are that high concentrations of the agent can be delivered to the local site and oral
rinses are easy to use. The principal disadvantages of this delivery system are that it
requires patient compliance, and drug pulses and concentration fluctuations may limit
efficacy. Rinses are also limited to supragingival and mucosal uses.

Oral irrigation   As with rinses, oral irrigation is relatively easy to use and can deliver
high concentrations of an agent to the local site. In addition, with training and newly
available equipment, it is possible to safely irrigate the subgingival area. This delivery
system does require greater patient dexterity and patient compliance, and also produces
the same fluctuations in drug concentration as noted for the oral rinses.

Controlled-release devices   "Controlled-release" refers to delivering active chemicals to a specified target at a rate and duration designed to accomplish the intended
effect. The advantages of such systems are *(1)* reproducible and prolonged constant rate
of delivery, *(2)* less frequent administration, and *(3)* greater patient compliance. As
with oral rinses, controlled-release systems offer advantages over systemic delivery in
that there are reduced side effects from the drugs, high concentrations are achieved at a
local site, and there is less patient variability. The primary disadvantage of such systems
is that they must be professionally applied. The most common types of controlled-
release devices are outlined in **Table 6.6**.

The most widely studied controlled-release device in periodontics has been **tetracycline fibers**. Although hollow fibers were initially used, the current fiber is a monolithic design in which tetracycline permeates an ethylene/vinyl acetate polymer. The fiber is inserted in the periodontal pocket and the moisture in the area dissolves the drug from the fiber surface as well as its interior as the polymer begins to dissolve. Tetracycline is initially released at a high rate, followed by relatively steady-state delivery for at least 10 days.

In order to maintain therapeutic levels of 4 to 8 μg/mL in gingival fluid for 10 days by means of systemic antibiotics, a total oral dose of 10 g is required. Tetracycline fibers with just 12.7 mg of active agent, when placed in periodontal pockets, have delivered between 643 to 1,590 μg/mL over a 10-day period.[1] The clinical benefits of subgingival controlled-release devices have recently been shown to be superior to scaling and root planing alone, and preliminary studies with tetracycline fibers also indicate some advantages over scaling and root planing alone in terms of the control of the subgingival microbiota. A variety of other controlled-release devices has been reported and are currently under investigation for the adjunctive treatment of periodontitis. This appears to be a promising therapeutic approach for localized areas of disease.

Summary

Topical application of antimicrobial agents is ideally suited for many of the microbial diseases that affect the oral cavity. These agents may be applied by oral rinsing, oral irrigation, or controlled-release devices. The selection of delivery system and agent depends on the target area to be treated and the therapeutic goal. Chapter 7 discusses the specific agents that may be used topically in the oral cavity.

References

1. Goodson, J.M. 1987. Drug delivery. *In* The American Academy of Periodontology. *Perspectives on Oral Antimicrobial Therapeutics*. Littleton, Mass.: PSG Publishing Co., pp. 61–78.
2. Goodson, J.M. 1989. Pharmacokinetic principles controlling efficacy of oral therapy. *J. Dent. Res.* 68:1625–1832.
3. Kydonieus, A.F. 1987. Fundamentals of transdermal drug delivery. *In* A.F. Kydonieus and B. Berner (eds.) *Transdermal Delivery of Drugs*. Boca Raton, Fla.: CRC Press, Inc., pp. 3–16.
4. Loesche, W.J. 1976. Chemotherapy of dental plaque infections. *Oral Sci. Rev.* 9:65–107.

CHAPTER 7

Topical Antimicrobial Agents: Individual Drugs

Kenneth S. Kornman, D.D.S., Ph.D.

Introduction

The selection of specific agents for use in topical antimicrobial therapy in the oral cavity should be based on the target area to be treated, the goals of therapy, and the delivery systems selected for use in the particular patient (see chapter 6). Controlled release of agents into the periodontal pocket often involves antibiotics such as tetracyclines or metronidazole; those agents are discussed in chapters 5 and 11. This chapter will focus on the topical agents that are routinely used as oral rinses and irrigants.

Topical antimicrobials directed at treating and controlling dental caries and gingivitis may be directed nonspecifically at supragingival plaque or may target specific bacterial components in the plaque.

Characteristics of topical agents

The selection of agents for topical use against caries and gingivitis should include consideration of toxicity, potency, and substantivity.

Toxicity   Although the oral mucous membranes may be easily irritated, all of the topical agents that are currently available commercially have low acute and chronic toxicity. These agents will not damage the oral mucosa with routine use, and extremely large volumes of these agents would have to be consumed systemically to achieve a fatal dose. Acute toxicity assessments of course do not include the unusual reactions such as allergic responses that have been reported for a small number of patients following treatment with either over-the-counter mouthwashes and toothpastes or chlorhexidine rinses.

Drug potency (see **Table 7.1**)   Potency refers to the concentration required to inhibit growth of specific types of bacteria. The lower the minimum inhibitory concen-

Table 7.1 Potency of commonly used topical antimicrobial agents*

Agent	Commercial form	Available concentration (μg/mL)	Gram-positive MIC 90 μg/mL†	Gram-negative MIC 90 μg/mL‡	Potency§	Reference
Cetylpyridinium chloride	Scope, Cepacol (Dow Chemical Co)	50	10,000	N/A	Low	1
Chlorhexidine	Peridex (Procter & Gamble)	1,200	32	4	Hi	2
Sanguinarine	Viadent	150	8	4	Hi	3
Sodium fluoride (daily rinse)	Fluorigard	500	2,048	256	Low	4
Thymol	Listerine	600	15,000	N/A	Low	5

*Adapted from Goodson (1989). [6]
†The concentration of drug required to inhibit growth of 90% of the gram-positive organisms tested.
‡The concentration of drug required to inhibit growth of 90% of the gram-negative organisms tested.
§Potency: Hi = MIC^{90} well below applied concentration.
　　　　Moderate = MIC^{90} close to applied concentration.
　　　　Low = MIC^{90} well above applied concentration.

tration (MIC) required, the higher the potency (see chapter 3). It is of course essential to relate inhibitory concentrations to the concentration of the drug that may be achieved in the target area. For topical application of antimicrobial agents, the actual concentration of the drug in the rinse represents the concentration available immediately to the supragingival plaque.

Substantivity Repeated studies have demonstrated that in vitro antibacterial activity of oral rinses is not a good predictor of in vivo antiplaque activity. To a great extent this discrepancy appears to be caused by fluctuations in concentration that result from intermittent application, that is, by rinses or irrigation of these agents (see chapter 6). For many years, potent antimicrobial agents were tested for antiplaque activity and demonstrated only minimum efficacy. The determining factor in a compound's antiplaque action appears to be retention in the oral cavity and release kinetics that allow prolonged antibacterial effects. This prolonged and effective availability of an agent is referred to as *substantivity.*

　　Substantivity actually involves three characteristics of the drug:

1. A relatively high proportion of the agent must be retained in the oral cavity. Agents with high substantivity bind by nonspecific attractive forces to a variety of oral sites.
2. The bound portion must be released over a reasonable time frame in order to maintain therapeutic levels. Thus, an agent with good substantivity will be bound and will release during a period of hours in order to prolong the effects. Some agents

(e.g., sanguinarine) will exhibit the first characteristic of binding but will not release in a manner that prolongs efficacy.

3. When the agent is released it must still be in an active form.

Substantivity therefore reduces the concentration fluctuations that result from intermittent drug application by means of rinses or irrigation. The impact of substantivity and other factors that determine the clearance of these agents from the oral cavity have been described in detail by Goodson.[6] Substantivity is of course of limited importance if controlled-release devices are used to maintain prolonged therapeutic levels of an agent.

Topical plaque-reduction agents

Development   Prior to the 1950s, when antibiotics began to dominate infection management, several reports indicated that topical antimicrobial agents might be effective in reducing plaque. Agents that showed some promise in limited clinical trials included phenol derivatives such as hexylresorcinol, surfactants such as sodium ricinoleate, heavy metals such as mercurials, and ammoniated compounds.

In the 1950s and 1960s, several antibiotics were used as topical preparations to inhibit plaque. At best they were marginally effective, and many results were contradictory. The realization that topical application of penicillin greatly increased the allergic response to this agent, and the fear that widespread topical use of medically important antibiotics might foster bacterial resistance and limit their usefulness in life-threatening situations, led to the discontinuation of locally applied antibiotics for reducing plaque (see chapter 6).

It is important to clearly identify the goal of antiplaque therapy. *Some agents may achieve statistically significant plaque reductions but have minimal to no clinical impact on disease.* Therefore, mechanical and chemical therapeutic approaches for gingivitis and the prevention of periodontitis may be deemed effective *(1)* if they prevent essentially all clinically detectable supragingival plaque, *(2)* if they alter plaque maturation, and most importantly *(3)* if they prevent clinical inflammation. *Plaque reduction per se does not demonstrate therapeutic efficacy.*

Three generations of antiplaque agents   Antimicrobial approaches to the prevention and treatment of gingivitis and subsequent prevention of periodontitis have focused on topical agents directed at nonspecific reduction or elimination of plaque. There are many topical compounds that inhibit or kill large numbers of oral bacteria, yet when they were tested in vivo, they did not prevent or treat gingivitis. These agents may be termed *first-generation agents.* They clearly demonstrate antibacterial capability in vitro but have minimal substantivity. First-generation agents have been available for many years and include a variety of compounds, ranging from topical antibiotics to peroxides. All mouthrinses that are currently available over the counter would be termed first-generation agents. There is no question that these agents are antibacterial, but they have limited efficacy in preventing or resolving signs of disease. When used in conjunction with conventional therapy, first-generation agents may give the clinical impression of efficacy; however, well-controlled clinical trails have demonstrated limited therapeutic value.

Second-generation agents have antibacterial activity plus proven substantivity. The recognition of the critical role of substantivity resulted from early studies with chlorhexidine. Although many excellent antibacterial agents had been evaluated for the prevention of plaque and gingivitis, chlorhexidine was the only compound to show consistently positive results. A series of studies in the early 1970s demonstrated that chlorhexidine was no different than several other compounds when tested in vitro for bacterial inhibition, but it was retained and slowly released in the oral cavity. Additional work confirmed that the unique efficacy of chlorhexidine was caused by its retention and release kinetics. For example, first-generation agents if used five to seven times daily may achieve efficacy comparable to chlorhexidine used only twice daily.

Chlorhexidine and its analogs are currently the only proven second-generation agents for prevention and control of gingivitis.

Third-generation agents are those agents that have selective effects on specific bacteria or bacterial products that are essential to disease development. The theoretical advantage of such agents over second-generation drugs is that they do not need to inhibit all plaque bacteria and therefore are more likely to be effective and safe in long-term usage. Chlorhexidine has some third-generation qualities in that *Actinomyces viscosus*, a key microorganism in the maturation of plaque that leads to gingivitis, is preferentially inhibited after rinsing or irrigation.[7] Earlier studies with enzymes that alter extracellular polysaccharides involved in plaque formation demonstrated the principles involved with third-generation agents. Although it is believed that increasing knowledge about bacterial adherence should allow the development of more agents with third-generation specificity, this direction has not yet produced practical approaches to therapy.

First-generation agents

Antibiotics

Systemic and topical applications of penicillin, tetracycline, polymyxin B, vancomycin, kanamycin, erythromycin, niddamycin, metronidazole, and spiromycin have been used to inhibit plaque and plaque-induced disease. In past evaluations, topical antibiotics in dentifrices or rinses have been unimpressive because of the administration of relatively low doses and the lack of prolonged effects from the antimicrobial agent. The potential for the development of bacterial resistance to important antibiotics and the development of patient hypersensitivity reactions to penicillin and a few other agents should limit the use of systemic antibiotics for plaque control purposes. These agents have therapeutic potential in the *treatment* of periodontitis when used systemically or with controlled release of antibiotics subgingivally. In general, antibiotics may hold great promise for specific bacterial diseases in the oral cavity but are inappropriate for routine control of supragingival plaque.

Quaternary ammonium compounds

These are cationic surface agents that are capable of reducing surface tension, absorbing to negatively charged surfaces, and disrupting membranes. These compounds are the active ingredients in several over-the-counter mouthwashes such as Scope® and Cepacol®.

Previous studies have demonstrated that quaternary ammonium compounds were effective at preventing the growth of plaque bacteria in vitro, but these results did not correlate with in vivo plaque inhibition. Clinical trials have been inconclusive because of the variability in results between studies.

Some of the apparent inconsistencies in results reported for the quaternary ammonium compounds may be explained by the observations of Bonesvoll and Gjermo,[8] relative to cetylpyridinium chloride (CPC). They noted that although twice as much CPC was retained in the mouth as chlorhexidine, the levels of CPC dropped quickly and continuously over the 12 hours after rinsing. Chlorhexidine, however, was retained for much longer and remained at stable levels even after 12 hours. This led to the hypothesis that quaternary ammonium compounds were less effective than chlorhexidine because of their limited substantivity. This hypothesis was tested by increasing the frequency of exposure. Rinses four times daily with quaternary ammonium compounds achieved a level of plaque prevention comparable to twice daily rinses with chlorhexidine.

Side effects with quaternary ammonium compounds have included both ulcerations and discomfort.

In general, quaternary ammonium compounds have shown a moderate degree of efficacy as antiplaque agents. They are rapidly absorbed to the tooth surface in a high concentration but are also rapidly released. Past antiplaque results with these agents are encouraging, although mucosal irritations have been reported in some trials and the lack of substantivity appears to limit clinical efficacy.

Phenolic compounds

These have a long history of use in the oral cavity as either mouthrinses or throat lozenges. Phenols in clinical trials have demonstrated mixed results. Several studies have evaluated the effectiveness of a commercial preparation (Listerine) of thymol and eucalyptol, methyl salicylate, benzoic acid, and boric acid, termed "essential oils." In general, these studies have noted statistically significant reductions in both plaque and gingivitis as compared to a placebo. The greatest effect of the agent appears to occur in the early stages of plaque formation in people who form large amounts of plaque. This agent has recently been recognized by the American Dental Association (ADA) as demonstrating efficacy in preventing plaque and gingivitis. This agent, therefore, appears to be capable of reducing plaque formation on a long-term basis, and its efficacy in combination with brushing is greater than brushing plus a placebo rinse. Its effect on gingivitis is statistically significant, but the clinical effect is limited and is consistent with its first-generation status. It is not yet known whether the degree of plaque and gingivitis inhibition caused by this agent is of long-term value in preventing periodontitis.

Sanguinarine

This is a benzophenanthradine alkaloid found in commercial mouthrinses (Viadent®) and toothpastes and has been reported to be potentially useful as a plaque-control agent. Reductions in plaque scores have been inconsistent between studies, and the agent has demonstrated a broad range of plaque effects. Similarly, the effects of sanguinarine on gingivitis have ranged from zero to statistically significant.

As discussed above, although this agent is retained in the oral cavity, it does not appear to have the release kinetics to allow prolonged efficacy between rinses. In general, previous studies indicate that sanguinarine is capable of some reduction and prevention of plaque and gingivitis. The degree of that effect appears to be modest and somewhat variable.

Fluorides

Fluorides have been widely used in dentistry for many years, and in terms of caries prevention they represent one of the most successful prevention agents in all of medicine. Evaluation of the specific mechanism of fluoride effect on the reduction of dental caries has led to the realization that fluoride may be of value in supragingival plaque control.

Stannous fluoride in concentrations exceeding 0.3% has shown some moderate ability to control plaque and gingivitis. Fluoride has a relatively low antibacterial potency. Although its release kinetics after application are reasonably good, so little of the agent is available for release that fluoride would still be best characterized as a first-generation agent.

Peroxides

Several peroxide-containing compounds are available or have been advocated as plaque-control agents. There are few well-controlled studies with these agents, and to date there appears to be no indication that peroxide compounds offer a therapeutic advantage over conventional home care in controlling plaque and gingivitis.

Prebrushing rinses

Extensive advertising in recent years has created a niche for plaque releasing agents (i.e., the prebrushing rinse). These products have been promoted as an aid to mechanical plaque removal, and the concept has appealed to consumers, as evidenced by strong sales. This market was developed by the advertising approach of Plax. This agent is not intended to be antibacterial but is a surfactant; that is, it is basically a soap that is supposed to help dislodge plaque so that it can be more efficiently removed. Early claims were based on one study, and subsequent studies have shown limited beneficial effects of this agent over rinsing with water alone.

A variety of other first-generation agents are available. In general, first-generation agents produce similar effects. With well-designed clinical studies, these agents will achieve statistically significant, although moderate, clinical effects. The in vitro antimicrobial potency of such agents does not predict their clinical usefulness.

Second-generation agents

At present, the only second-generation antiplaque/antigingivitis agents (i.e., those with antimicrobial activity plus evidence of substantivity) are chlorhexidine and its analogs.

Chlorhexidine

The most promising topical agent for reducing dental plaque and treating gingivitis is clearly **chlorhexidine gluconate**. This agent has been widely used in ophthalmic and skin preparations and has demonstrated a high degree of effectiveness and low toxicity when used topically. Extensive human studies have shown that, in the absence of mechanical plaque control, a 1-minute mouthrinse twice daily with 10 mL of 0.2% chlorhexidine gluconate completely inhibited plaque formation for up to 40 days and produced an 85% to 90% reduction in tooth-adherent bacteria. Subsequent studies have shown that approximately 30% of the agent is retained in the mouth after rinsing, where it is active in inhibiting bacterial absorption and growth. Chlorhexidine is slowly released such that antibacterial activity persists in saliva for several hours after rinsing. In fact, early studies indicate that up to half of the retained chlorhexidine is still present after 2 hours.

Mathematical models of the oral clearance of chlorhexidine[6] in different subjects suggest that the agent may be above antibacterial levels in saliva for between 3 to 8 hours after an early-morning rinse. These same models indicate that with the reduction in saliva flow normally observed during sleep, a chlorhexidine rinse at bedtime may provide persistent antibacterial levels in saliva for well over 12 hours.[6]

Long-term studies in both humans and dogs indicate that some plaque regrowth occurs after a few months of regular chlorhexidine use. Because certain oral bacteria such as *Streptococcus* and *Capnocytophaga* sp. are relatively resistant to the agent, plaque control by means of chlorhexidine rinses with no other oral hygiene measures for extended periods of time may not be practical. The regrowth of plaque dominated by

---

Table 7.2 Sample prescription for chlorhexidine gluconate rinse

---

Rx: Peridex 0.12%

Dispense: Three (3) bottles

Label: Rinse with 1 capful for 30 seconds every morning and
           every evening after brushing teeth

           Do not rinse mouth with water after using Peridex

---

these two microorganisms is probably a positive result of chlorhexidine, and this type of plaque is unlikely to be associated with either gingivitis or periodontitis. In addition, studies that have evaluated chlorhexidine as an adjunct to toothbrushing have generally achieved such good plaque control by mechanical means alone that the incremental effect of chlorhexidine plus toothbrushing could not be adequately evaluated.

Recent long-term studies using 0.12% chlorhexidine have confirmed the value of this agent as an oral rinse for preventing and treating gingival inflammation. Chlorhexidine in the form of Peridex (Procter & Gamble) is approved by both the U.S. Food and Drug Administration (FDA) and the ADA for use in treating gingival inflammation and associated bleeding. It is available by prescription only (see **Table 7.2**) and is currently the only agent approved by the FDA as a treatment for gingivitis.

Side effects Chlorhexidine has been used widely as a topical disinfectant for more than 25 years. During this period, reports of adverse reactions associated with applications of chlorhexidine to intact skin, mucous membranes, and traumatic or surgical wounds have been few. Long-term effects of animal feeding and topical human use show that absorption through the alimentary mucosa or through the skin is negligible. The incidence of hypersensitivity is low, but gingival hypersensitivity reactions to Peridex have been reported in a small number of individuals.

Oral use of chlorhexidine has been associated with **staining** of the teeth, tongue, and anterior restorations. Staining varies greatly among individuals and appears to reach substantial levels only in about 15% of the subjects studied. Staining appears to be most prominent in patients who show stains before chlorhexidine use and in individuals who heavily consume tanin-containing substances, such as tea and red wine. Staining of exposed cementum appears to be more common than staining of enamel surfaces. Anterior restorations with rough surfaces or margins are also more likely to stain. Because the stain is entirely extrinsic, it can be removed by polishing with minimum difficulty in most patients. Patients who are prone to staining and patients with cementum staining will require more time for stain removal and may benefit from the judicious use of an air-pressure polisher such as the Prophyjet.

Although chlorhexidine is extremely effective in plaque prevention, some individuals may show a slight increase in **supragingival calculus**, especially on the lingual surfaces of mandibular anterior teeth. This calculus appears to have a different

---

Table 7.3   Common uses of chlorhexidine rinses

Adjunctive supragingival plaque control

- In the management of recurrent or persistent gingivitis
- Following oral surgery/periodontal surgery
- Following crown preparation and during period that provisional restorations are worn
- For physically or mentally handicapped patients

Treatment and control of oral mucosal infections

- Rampant caries
- Gingivitis in immunocompromised patients (e.g., HIV gingivitis) (see chapter 18)
- Prevention and control of mild candidiasis in immunocompromised patients (see chapter 18)
- Aphthous ulcers

Adjunctive control of bacterial recolonization

- In association with treatment of periodontitis
- In association with systemic controlled-release antibiotic treatment of subgingival bacteria

---

composition from routine calculus deposits, is easily removed, and appears to have no harmful effects.

Some patients will experience transient **taste alteration** following chlorhexidine rinses. This effect can be minimized by instructing the patient to rinse after meals and to avoid rinsing with water after the chlorhexidine.

Uses   Chlorhexidine has been studied and used for many purposes, but in general the most common uses of chlorhexidine rinses fall into three categories (see **Table 7.3**). The primary use involves rinsing as an adjunct to supragingival plaque control. This is appropriate for the management of recurrent or persistent gingivitis. For example, maintenance patients who continue to show gingival bleeding in spite of regular professional supportive therapy and reinforcement of oral hygiene practices have been shown to benefit from chlorhexidine rinses. This agent is now routinely used as a rinse after oral surgery and periodontal surgery. The agent should be used for a minimum of 2 weeks after surgery, and there are some indications that additional benefits may result from even longer usage.

Although chlorhexidine rinses are effective with and without the concomitant use of periodontal dressings, it is common practice today in many cases of periodontal surgery to prescribe chlorhexidine rinses instead of placing a dressing. In this situation the chlorhexidine keeps the surgical area clean, promotes wound healing, and facilitates overall plaque control at a time when the patient may be less attentive to home-care hygiene.

This agent has also been shown to provide tissue benefits following tooth preparation for crown-and-bridge procedures (see chapter 15). The benefits appear to be similar to those observed following periodontal surgery.

Use of chlorhexidine for supragingival plaque control has also been advocated for physically or mentally handicapped patients. The agent may be applied in these cases by means of a tooth sponge rather than rinsing.

A second general use of chlorhexidine rinses is in the treatment and control of oral infections. Although fluoride is the most commonly used chemical agent for caries control, chlorhexidine is a potent and specific agent for the control of *Streptococcus mutans*, the microbial cause of dental caries. Chlorhexidine appears to be especially effective for controlling rampant caries in some patients. As discussed in chapter 18, chlorhexidine is a very useful agent in managing oral infections in immunocompromised patients. Gingivitis and mild candidiasis in these patients are generally responsive to chlorhexidine therapy. One of the most rewarding uses of chlorhexidine is in the treatment of aphthous ulcers. These intraoral lesions that are found on movable mucosa respond rapidly to frequent topical application of chlorhexidine. This may be applied by a cotton swab or rinse.

Chlorhexidine rinses have been shown to be beneficial in reducing bacterial repopulation following subgingival therapy. *Oral rinses do not reach the subgingival compartment;* however, with either mechanical or chemical treatment of the subgingival bacteria, chlorhexidine rinses improve the clinical outcome. This effect is most likely caused by interference with recolonization of the subgingival area.

Topical treatment of caries

Bacterial studies in recent years have strongly implicated *S. mutans* as a causative agent in human dental caries. Antimicrobial treatment can therefore be directed at suppressing or reducing this organism. Because the tooth surface is essentially the only reservoir for *S. mutans*, and because the organism does not appear to be readily transmitted, disinfection of tooth surfaces could theoretically result in a prolonged elimination of *S. mutans* from the oral cavity. This treatment effect is plausible because recolonization of the teeth will occur primarily from salivary bacteria, which would originate from nontooth reservoirs.

Fluoride

At present, the most promising agent for disinfecting the tooth surface appears to be fluoride. This approach, unlike nonspecific treatment, requires an intensive topical regimen in conjunction with excavation of existing carious lesions that might reseed bacteria to other sites. Because cariogenic bacteria can penetrate the tooth surface, disinfection might have to be repeated in order to destroy organisms that can grow out of the tooth and reinfect the area. Unfortunately, there are no firm guidelines for this

---

Table 7.4   Topical fluoride for treating rampant caries

---

1. Excavate carious lesions and place permanent restorations.
2. After restorations are placed, provide 1 week of intensive fluoride therapy: stannous fluoride 0.4% gel in application trays. Apply twice daily for 4 min. Expectorate excess gel and do not eat, drink, or rinse for 30 min following application.
3. Repeat fluoride treatment for 1 week following every 6-month recall.
4. If new carious lesions are detected, repeat steps 1 and 2 above.

---

treatment approach. Loesche[9] suggested one protocol (see **Table 7.4**) for topical antibacterial treatment of dental caries.

Chlorhexidine

Chlorhexidine is highly specific against *S. mutans* and has been shown to be an effective agent in treating rampant caries. After all carious lesions are excavated and either provisional or permanent restorations have been placed, chlorhexidine should be prescribed for 6 weeks. The patient should also receive oral hygiene instructions and counseling to reduce intake of a cariogenic food. Ideally, the patient's saliva should be monitored for *S. mutans* levels. This can be done in the private office by means of commercially available test kits. If microbial testing is performed, chlorhexidine should be used until *S. mutans* counts are reduced.

Summary

Modest plaque control using topical antimicrobials may be achieved by means of over-the-counter mouthrinses, of which Listerine is currently accepted by the ADA. Treatment and control of gingivitis, treatment of microbial oral infections, and adjunctive use in various conditions, including periodontitis, appear to require greater efficacy, which is currently available in the form of chlorhexidine rinses, which are FDA and ADA approved for control of gingival inflammation. Use of chlorhexidine requires an understanding of the agent and how to manage potential side effects.

References

1. Dzink, J.L., and Socransky, S.S. 1985. Comparative in vitro activity of sanguinarine against oral microbial isolates. *Antimicrob. Agents Chemother.* 27:663–665.

2. Emilson, C.G. 1977. Susceptibility of various microorganisms to chlorhexidine. *Scand. J. Dent. Res.* 85:255–265.

3. Evans, R.T., Baker, P.J., Coburn, R.A., and Genco, R.J. 1977. In vitro antiplaque effects of antiseptic phenols. *J. Periodontol.* 48:156–162.

4. Mandell, R.L. 1983. Sodium fluoride susceptibilities of suspected periodontopathic bacteria. *J. Dent. Res.* 62:706–708.

5. Tanzer, J.M., Slee, A.M., Kamay, B., and Sheer, E.R. 1979. In vitro evaluation of seven cationic detergents as antiplaque agents. *Antimicrob. Agents Chemother.* 15:408–414.

6. Goodson, J.M. 1989. Pharmacokinetic principles controlling efficacy of oral therapy. *J. Dent. Res.* 68:1625–1632.

7. Brownstein, C.N., Briggs, S.D., Schweiter, K.L., Briner, W.W., and Kornman, K.S. 1990. Irrigation with chlorhexidine to resolve naturally occurring gingivitis: A methodologic study. *J. Clin. Periodontol.* (In press.)

8. Bonesvoll, P., and Gjermo, P. 1978. A comparison between chlorhexidine and some quaternary ammonium compounds with regard to retention, salivary concentration and plaque inhibiting effect in the human mouth after mouthrinses. *Arch. Oral Biol.* 23:289–294.

9. Loesche, W.J. 1982. *Dental Caries: A Treatable Infection.* Springfield, Ill.: Charles C Thomas, Publisher.

Further reading

Löe, H., and Kleinman, D.V. (eds.) 1986. *Dental Plaque Control Measures and Oral Hygiene Practices.* Washington, D.C.: IRL Press.

CHAPTER 8

✓ Antifungal and Antiviral Agents

Kenneth S. Kornman, D.D.S., Ph.D.

A high incidence of oral fungal infections in patients on immunosuppressive therapy and in patients who have tested positive for the human immunodeficiency virus has greatly increased the dental use of antifungal agents.

Most fungi are completely resistant to the action of antibacterial drugs. Although the fungal cell wall is very different from that of mammalian cells and it should be possible to design drugs based on these differences, currently there are very few substances available that are effective against fungi pathogenic for humans. Unfortunately, most of these agents are also relatively toxic for humans. This chapter will focus on antifungal drugs that may be used topically. Systemic use of some agents will also be noted because this approach should be considered if topical agents are ineffective. The uses of antifungal and antiviral drugs in the management of immunocompromised patients are discussed in chapter 18.

Topical antifungal agents

Topical antifungal agents for use in the oral cavity can be divided into two categories: *polyenes* and *imidazoles*.

Polyenes **Nystatin** has been the most widely used topical antifungal drug. It is a polyene macrolide that has no effect on bacteria but inhibits many fungi, including *Candida* sp. The mode of action is by disruption of the fungal membrane. Although resistance does not routinely develop, drug-resistant strains of *Candida* will occur. Nystatin is poorly soluble in water and is not absorbed by the skin, mucous membranes, or gastrointestinal tract. Almost all nystatin applied in the oral cavity is excreted in the feces, with no significant blood or tissue levels achieved.

Nystatin is available for intraoral use as an oral suspension or as a pastille (Mycostatin). The pastilles are troches that contain 200,000 units of nystatin and are designed to slowly dissolve in the mouth. Levels of nystatin sufficient to inhibit growth of

Table 8.1 Antifungal agents for treatment for oral candidiasis

Agent	Available form	Recommended use
Nystatin	Topical: Mycostatin pastilles	Dissolve one pastille 5 times daily for 14 d
	Nystatin Oral Suspension	Swish with 4–6 mL (400,000–600,000 units) 4 times daily for 14 d. Retain in mouth for 2 min before swallowing. Continue treatment for at least 48 h after symptoms have disappeared.
Clotrimazole	Topical: Mycelex troches	Dissolve 1 troche 5 times daily for 14 d
Ketoconazole	Systemic: Nizoral	One tablet (200 mg) daily for 14 d
Fluconazole	Systemic: Diflucan	Two (100-mg) tablets the first day then one tablet daily for a minimum total treatment of 14 d

Candida albicans persist in the saliva for 2 hours after oral dissolution of two pastilles. The usual adult dosage for oral candidiasis is one to two pastilles dissolved slowly five times daily for 10 to 14 days. Therapy should not be interrupted during that period of time unless adverse effects are noted, and therapy should continue for at least 48 hours after disappearance of oral symptoms. Although nystatin has a generally unpleasant taste, the anise-flavored pastilles are relatively well accepted by patients. See **Table 8.1** for recommended use of nystatin.

Imidazoles   Synthetic imidazole antifungals inhibit fungi by blocking the synthesis of cell membrane components. These agents are available primarily as clotrimazole, miconazole, ketoconazole, and fluconazole (see **Table 8.1**). **Clotrimazole** is the primary agent in this group for topical oral use. It is available as 10-mg troches (Mycelex) to be used five times daily for 14 days to suppress oral candidiasis. After use of one troche, concentrations sufficient to inhibit most strains of *Candida* sp. persist in the saliva for up to 3 hours. Repeated oral dosing every 3 hours maintains salivary levels above the minimum inhibitory concentration of most strains of *Candida*.

Miconazole is available in vaginal and dermatologic topical preparations (Monistat) and is not intended for topical oral use. **Ketoconazole** is a relatively recent addition to the imidazole agents. It is also the first antifungal effective in systemic mycoses that can be taken by mouth. This agent is appropriate for treating oral candidiasis in patients where topical antifungal therapy has not resolved the symptoms or when there have been frequent recurrences. One of the advantages of ketoconazole is that it is administered once daily in tablet form (Nizoral) for 7 to 14 days. As with all systemic antifungal agents, ketoconazole has toxic effects, including nausea, vomiting, skin rashes, and alteration of synthesis of adrenal steroids. Serious side effects occur infrequently. Anorexia, nausea, and vomiting occur in 3% to 10% of patients and can usually be reduced by taking the drug with food. Interference with steroid synthesis may be a problem with prolonged use (6 weeks). Absorption of the drug requires an acidic pH in the stomach, which may limit its efficacy in patients who have achlorhydria or who are taking antacids or histamine antagonists.

A new imidazole, **fluconazole** (Diflucan), appears to have promise in persistent cases of oral candidiasis and has the advantage of once-daily dosing. Although early reports suggest that this agent provides an outstanding treatment outcome, only limited data are available at this time.

Antiviral agents

The dramatic increase in chronic viral infections, including herpes and AIDS, has fostered extensive development efforts in the area of antiviral drugs. Because viruses depend entirely on the metabolic processes of the host cell, chemicals that inhibit viral replication also inhibit some host cell function and frequently possess substantial toxicity. This has greatly complicated the search for effective antiviral agents that possess minimal toxicity. In addition, because viral replication usually reaches a maximum just before clinical symptoms appear, it is difficult to time the effect of administrating antiviral drugs.

The most widely used agent for herpetic lesions is **acyclovir** (Zovirax). Acyclovir is metabolized to an active product that inhibits herpes virus DNA polymerase. Topical application of 5% acyclovir ointment has been shown to shorten the healing time and reduce the pain when applied early to lesions in primary genital herpes. Topical application has a limited effect on recurrent genital lesions. Oral acyclovir in doses of 200 mg five times daily also exhibits good results in primary genital herpes. When taken prophylactically for extended periods of time, it can reduce the frequency and severity of recurrent genital lesions. Patients who have stopped using the drug have reported a rebound effect with increased frequency of episodes.

Recurrent oral herpetic lesions may also respond to oral acyclovir therapy, but topical application of acyclovir ointment in the oral cavity appears to have limited efficacy.

Long-term therapy (chronic suppressive therapy, see **Table 8.2**) generally involves 200 mg of acyclovir five times daily for the first 3 days and then 200 mg of acyclovir two to four times daily for 6 to 9 months. This approach is reasonable for patients who experience six or more severe recurrent episodes per year. Chronic suppressive therapy has been shown to significantly reduce the number of episodes. In general, drug-resistant strains have not been found except in immunocompromised patients who have received multiple doses of therapy. Chronic suppressive therapy should be stopped after 6 to 9 months. Although extensive development work is underway in this area, the introduction of new antiviral drugs will be slow.

Table 8.2   Chronic acyclovir therapy to suppress recurrent herpetic episodes

---

Acyclovir (Zovirax) 200-mg tablets:

- Take 1 tablet 5 times daily for the first 3 d, then
- Take 1 tablet 2 to 4 times daily for 6 mo
- Reevaluate after 6 mo and discontinue therapy
- Chronic suppressive therapy may be reinstituted if patient is stable and has decreased incidence of herpetic episodes after stopping therapy but then the episodes reactivate months or years later

---

Further reading

Bodey, G.P. 1988. Topical and systemic antifungal agents. *Med. Clin. North Am.* 72:637–659.

Epstein, J.B. 1989. Oral and pharyngeal candidiasis. Topical agents for management and prevention. *Postgrad. Med.* 85:257–258, 263–265, 268–269.

Meunier, F. 1987. Prevention and mycoses in immunocompromised patients. *Rev. Infect. Dis.* 9:408–416.

Reines, E.D., and Gross, P.A. 1988. Antiviral agents. *Med. Clin. North Am.* 72:691–715.

PART 3

ADVERSE REACTIONS

CHAPTER 9

Allergic and Other Sensitivity Reactions

Larry J. Peterson, D.D.S., M.S.

Advances in knowledge   The study of allergy and immunology has advanced tremendously in the past several decades. A new era in the understanding of allergy was born in 1967 when Dr. Ishizaka described IgE, the class of antibody (immunoglobulin) associated with anaphylaxis. For decades before this time, traceable back to the late 19th and early 20th centuries, investigators had been concerned primarily with the immunologic bases of infection and vaccine. In the early 20th century, interest turned to allergic reactions. It was not until the mid-1960s that investigators began to understand more clearly the basis of immunologic reactions. The achievements in the field since have been phenomenal. A better understanding of patient sensitivity and hypersensitivity to selected substances has opened doors to safer patient management.

Allergy vs. immunity   Clemens Freiherr von Pirquet coined the term "allergy" in the early 20th century. He used it to describe any altered reaction of the immune system, whether helpful or harmful. In the context of immunology today, *immunity* is thought of as protective and implies enhanced resistance, whereas *allergy* is thought of as harmful and suggests increased susceptibility to a specific substance.

Elements of the immune response

Antibodies and allergens

In the allergic response, self recognizes nonself and a series of complicated immunologic reactions are initiated. An antibody, usually of the IgE class, attaches to either a mast cell or a basophil, making it ready to receive allergens.

An allergen, possibly an inhalant such as grass, pollen, mold, a food or drug fragment, or a high-molecular-weight molecule, attaches to the antibody fixed to the mast cell or basophil. This attachment triggers a number of cellular and immunologic reactions.

Inflammation

An allergic reaction produces inflammation, which is a basic response of the body to injury. The inflammatory response includes a complex series of events, which involves *(1)* receptor cells, including the basophil, mast cell, eosinophil, and neutrophil; *(2)* chemical mediators, including histamine and SRS-A; and *(3)* larger molecules and enzymes found in the complement system. The role of chemical mediators has not been clearly defined. They are believed protective, although their release can cause the patient to be acutely symptomatic, suffering an allergic episode. In addition to the chemical mediators that mast cells and basophils release, other mediators in the complement system augment the efficiency of immunologic function. The complement system aids in the removal of certain nonself materials and in the production of inflammation.

Immunoglobulins

Five classes of immunoglobulins, or antibodies, are known. These are IgG, IgA, IgM, IgD, and IgE. Immunoglobulins are usually thought to play mostly protective roles in humans. However, their exact roles have not been fully described, and certainly while most properties seem to be protective, some properties are obviously harmful. The IgE is believed to play an allergic role in the organism because it is the primary antibody in type 1 immunologic reactions. IgG subclass IV, a homocytotropic (cell-bound) antibody, is also suspected to be important in allergic reactions.

Specialized cells

Lymphocytes and macrophages   Several types of cells maintain the body's immunologic response. Lymphocytes, classified as T lymphocytes **(T cells)** and B lymphocytes **(B cells)**, are crucial to this function. T cells are involved as helpers, suppressors, and killers. B cells are the progenitors of plasma cells, which synthesize immunoglobulins. In their interactions with macrophage cells, which help process antigenic material, B cells lead to the production of specific antibodies. T cells either promote or suppress the production. Lymphokines, which arise from T cells, are messenger proteins that facilitate immunologic responses and other cellular interactions.

Basophils and mast cells   Basophils and mast cells are rich sources of mediators such as histamine, slow-reacting substance of anaphylaxis (SRS-A), eosinophil chemotactic factor of anaphylaxis (ECF-A), platelet-activating factor (PAF), bradykinin, and prostaglandins. IgE antibodies will fix to either basophils or mast cells. It is the attachment of the antigen (allergen) to the antibody IgE that triggers the eventual release of these mediators. Mast cells, basophils, and the IgE system are associated with the immediate hypersensitivity or type 1 reaction. They do not play prominent roles in other types of immunologic reactions.

Eosinophils and leukocytes   Levels of eosinophils are frequently elevated during acute allergic reactions. They can be found in the blood, nasal secretions, and sputum and seem to play a role in combating the effects of certain chemical mediators, including SRS-A arylsulfatase. Polymorphonuclear leukocytes (PMNs) also participate in some immunologic reactions.

Types of immunologic responses

Sensitive vs. allergic   We often call all drug reactions or other sensitivity or hypersensitivity reactions allergic. But allergic reactions are just one type of immunologic reaction (see **Table 9.1**). **Allergic reactions are of the type 1 class.** Immunologic reactions are broadly classified into four types.

Types of cellular reactions: overview   **Type 1** reactions are immediate immunologic reactions, usually allergic reactions, and usually mediated by IgE or homocytotropic IgG. **Type 2** reactions are *cytotoxic* reactions, where an IgG or IgM antibody reacts with cell membranes or antigens associated with cell membranes. **Type 3** reactions are *immune complex* reactions, where an antigen and antibody combine together to form an immune complex that deposits in the walls of blood vessels, the kidneys, or other selected areas. **Type 4** reactions are *delayed hypersensitivity* or *cell-mediated reactions,* where cells interact directly with antigens.

Allergic reactions are only those type 1 reactions mediated by IgE or similar homocytotropic (cell-bound) immunoglobulins. When caring for patients we deal with many reactions of types 2 to 4. Rather than calling these reactions "allergic," as is most often done, we should call them "immunologic."

Type 1: immediate hypersensitivity

Symptoms   Type 1 reactions to drugs predominantly affect the skin and respiratory

Table 9.1   Types of hypersensitivity

Class	Name	Indicator
Type 1	Immediate	IgE, rarely IgG$_4$
Type 2	Cytotoxic	IgG, IgM, rarely IgA
Type 3	Immune complex	IgG (usually)
Type 4	Delayed	Cellular

system. Severe reactions can provoke rash, urticaria, angioedema, respiratory distress and wheezing, and even anaphylaxis and shock. Anaphylaxis is an extreme allergic reaction that can lead to respiratory and cardiovascular collapse.

Agents   **Penicillin** and **horse serum sensitivity** can cause classic examples of a type 1 reaction. Other drugs and substances, including allergens used for immunotherapy, xenogenic sera, insulin, the haptene metabolites of simple chemical drugs, and certain proteins of biologic products, can also be involved in immediate hypersensitivity type 1 reactions.

Type 2: cytotoxic reactions

Reaction   Cytotoxic reactions are complement-dependent and usually involve IgG or IgM antibodies. An antibody-drug-complement complex fixes to a circulating blood cell, causing cell lysis. A **blood type mismatch** is an example of a cytotoxic reaction.

Mechanisms   There are three mechanisms of cytotoxic blood reactions. In the first, the drug fixes to a cell membrane and an antibody attaches to the drug to form an antibody-antigen complex. Complement is activated and cell lysis occurs. Penicillin-induced immunohemolytic anemia is this type of cytotoxic reaction.

In the second mechanism, the drug, antibody, and complement form a complex *before* attaching to a cell wall and cell lysis. This is the reaction that results in direct Coombs-positive anti-immune hemolytic anemia, leukopenia, and thrombocytopenia after exposure to certain drugs, including quinidine and sulfonamides.

The third mechanism occurs when the red blood cell membrane is modified by a drug, causing the cell to absorb protein nonspecifically. Cytotoxic cellular destruction results.

Type 3: immune complex reactions

Reaction   Immunologic sensitivities can be mediated by immune complex reactions. Serum sickness is a reaction of this type and may be caused by heterologous serum or a heptenic drug determinant such as penicillin. The reaction is systemic and can involve multiple organ systems. **Complement-dependent vasculitis** often results, with immune complexes depositing along endothelial surfaces of blood vessels to stimulate inflammation and vascular wall damage.

Symptoms   Symptoms of serum sickness, while not as immediately devastating as anaphylactic reactions, are quite serious. They include fever, arthralgia, lymphadenopathy, and rash. Dermatologic manifestations include erythema multiforme, urticaria, which may persist for weeks, and angioedema. A latent period of several days usually passes after the initial administration of a drug before enough antibody to provoke symptoms is produced.

Agents   Other drugs and substances that can invoke immune complex reactions are foreign sera, penicillin, sulfonamides, thiouracils, diphenylhydantoin, aminosalicylic acid, and streptomycin.

Type 4: delayed hypersensitivity

Reaction   The allergic contact dermatitis that can develop from the use of **topical penicillin or other topical drugs** is a cell-mediated, delayed hypersensitivity process. T cells interact directly with antigens.

Agents   Substances that can cause a delayed hypersensitivity reaction include topical antibiotics, topical antihistamines, topical local anesthetics, and certain additives found in topical medications, including parabens and lanolin. Patch testing can help to establish the agent causing these reactions. However, testing is not always productive and the cause may go undetected.

Immunologic reactions to drugs: Overview

Incidence

Until World War II, serum sickness was the most common allergic drug reaction observed. With the introduction of sulfonamides in the 1930s, more allergic drug reactions were seen. With the increased availability of small molecular weight drugs and foreign proteins, the incidence of drug sensitization seems to have increased.

The risk for developing an allergic reaction to most drugs is approximately 2% to 3%. Adverse drug reactions as a whole, which includes both allergic and nonallergic responses, are experienced by approximately 10% to 15% of *hospitalized* patients. Adults predominate in this group. Less than 7% of the adverse reactions are life-threatening.

Examples of common drug reactions

Potential sources of drug reactions and possible allergic problems used by the dentist in patient care are: penicillin and other antibiotics; local anesthetics of the ester type and related drugs; adjunctive vasoconstrictors, such as epinephrine; and other preparations including sedatives, antihistamines, and analgesics.

Clinical vs. pharmacological effects   The clinical manifestations of drug allergy differ from the pharmacological effects of the drug. While in most cases pharmacological effects are beneficial, clinical manifestations of drug allergy may be harmful to the body. The clinical response in humans cannot always be predicted from animal tests. Drug allergy involves a small portion of the population and is usually restricted to a limited number of syndromes. Clinically, the patient may develop numerous symptoms, including:

- Urticaria
- Angioedema
- Rash
- Asthma

- Systemic anaphylaxis
- Fever
- Adenopathy
- Pulmonary infiltrates

Prior exposure

Allergic and immunologic drug reactions are fascinating and frequently pose a significant clinical challenge to the dental practitioner. In many cases, the patient may have been exposed to a drug during earlier treatment and had no reaction. After a patient develops sensitivity, and the drug is reintroduced into his or her system, the immunologic response may be immediate or may appear after several days. The risk of developing an immunologic response to a drug exists at doses below the therapeutic range. **In some cases very tiny exposures to a drug can trigger an allergic response.**

A patient must have been exposed to an agent at least once before in order to develop an allergic sensitivity to it. Medically it is almost impossible to have an allergic reaction to one's first dose of penicillin. After a patient develops sensitivity to a drug and it is reintroduced into his or her system, the immunologic response can be immediate or delayed for several days. The response should resolve when the drug is withdrawn.

In some cases a patient may have been unknowingly exposed to a drug. For example, a small amount of penicillin naturally occurring in milk can cause sensitivity to develop undetected.

Heredity

Patients may inherit the tendency to become allergic to drugs. On the other hand, patients experiencing an allergic drug reaction do not necessarily have a history of allergy or atopy. While speculative, there is evidence for genetic influence on drug metabolism, and patients who metabolize drugs more slowly are believed more likely to develop allergic drug reaction.

Sensitivity testing

It is important to understand the basis of the patient's allergic reaction both for deciding whether to continue antibiotic treatment and for managing the reaction itself.

Inconsistent reliability   Immunologic testing to confirm sensitivity or allergy to a drug is not always reliable. Two factors contribute to this:

1. The immunologic bases for many allergic drug reactions have not been clearly defined.
2. The patient may be reacting to a metabolite of a drug, or to its dye or capsular material, rather than, or in addition to, the drug itself.

Consultation with a specialist   Because of the uncertainties in interpretation of test results, it is best to consult an allergist or immunologist to clarify the status of a patient with suspected drug sensitivity. The tools for determining the nature of allergic drug reactions are not readily available to all practitioners.

Reliable tests

Systemic sensitivity can be indicated for certain large molecular substances including horse serum, insulin, and ACTH. Tests for only a few low-molecular-weight drugs, such as penicillin, are developed enough to yield fairly reliable results. Few drugs responsible for hematologic reactions can be tested reliably.

Positive skin tests are helpful because they verify sensitivity. But only in the case of penicillin are negative skin tests significant. In most other cases a negative result could mean the component causing sensitivity was not represented in the sample tested.

The most conclusive test of sensitivity is to rechallenge the patient, but the risk is usually not justified. An exception is patch testing for agents suspected responsible for an allergic eczematous contact dermatitis.

Types of tests

In vivo immunologic tests include immediate skin tests, delayed skin tests, patch testing, and skin window techniques. **In vitro** tests test for IgE, IgG, and IgM antibodies and for sensitized lymphocytes. IgE antibodies are detectable with leukocyte histamine release, rat mast cell degranulation, sensitized human and monkey lung histamine release, RAST, and total IgE level. Tests for circulating antibodies and Rosette testing locate IgG and IgM antibodies. Tests for determination of sensitized lymphocytes include lymphocyte transformation assays and macrophage inhibition determinations.

Penicillin hypersensitivity

Penicillin hypersensitivity frequently is a major roadblock in the management of dental infections. The widely used drug **can cause almost every known type of sensitivity reaction.**

Incidence   It has been suggested that some type of adverse reaction occurs in 3% of penicillin users.

Determinants

Penicilloic acid, a metabolic degradation product, is the major determinant of type 1 reactions and is often primarily responsible for late urticarial reactions and other skin eruptions. Anaphylaxis and immediate urticaria or angioedema can be caused by other antigenic determinants, known as minor determinants. These have not yet been fully characterized but seem to be responsible for severe types of immediate allergic reactions such as anaphylaxis. The source of the protein carriers for this haptenic determinant has not been clearly defined. The natures of the antigenic determinants in types 2, 3, and 4 reactions to penicillin are not known.

Manifestations

Skin eruptions   **The most common manifestation of penicillin allergy is a diffuse erythematous or morbilliform skin eruption.** Allergic-contact dermatitis may be seen after the topical use of penicillin.

Anaphylaxis   Anaphylaxis occurs in about one in 10,000 patients using penicillin, accounting for approximately 300 deaths per year in the United States. When urticaria or angioedema appear less than an hour after administration, anaphylaxis should be considered. More severe anaphylactic reactions have systemic involvement and compromise breathing. Urticaria that begins days to weeks after penicillin is administered seems to have less serious implications and in some cases may disappear even if penicillin treatment is continued.

Type 3 reactions   Immune complex–mediated reactions such as serum sickness will occur occasionally, as will immunohemolytic anemia, which can complicate high-dose intravenous therapy.

Cessation of symptoms

When penicillin is discontinued, the drug reaction subsides. In some cases, urticarial rash may persist for many months and may be triggered occasionally by trace amounts of penicillin found in dietary milk. Avoidance of milk products may be helpful in these cases.

Cautions

Concurrent infectious processes can produce an exanthematous eruption that mimics a penicillin sensitivity, possibly causing erroneous diagnosis of penicillin allergy. Awareness of this is especially important when penicillin is given to children with viral or streptococcal respiratory infections. There is some cross-reactivity and cross-allergy between penicillin and the cephalosporins. When cephalosporins are started in a patient with a history of penicillin sensitivity, caution should be exercised.

Diagnosis with skin testing

Detection of determinants   Skin testing to detect IgE antibodies to major and minor determinants can be useful in the diagnosis of penicillin allergy. Penicilloyl-Polylysine (manufactured by several pharmaceutical companies) is marketed to test for the major determinants of this hypersensitivity. A minor determinant mixture is not commercially available, but using penicillin G at 10,000 units/mL serum has correlated well with minor determinants. It is the currently recommended method.

Interpretation of results   If the major determinant test is positive, there is a high correlation with skin manifestations such as rash and urticaria. If the minor determinant test is positive, the risk of anaphylaxis is very high. Negative skin test reactions to both major and minor determinants suggest that the patient is probably not allergic to penicillin.

Hemagglutination detects serum IgG and IgM antibodies. IgG antibody may function as a "blocking antibody" and have a protective function. Both IgG and IgM antibodies may produce a type 2 hemolytic anemia if penicillin is given in high dosages intravenously.

When to test   Sufficient controversy surrounds this still-developing area so that a clear directive of when to test cannot be given. In the opinion of the author, the best time to do penicillin skin testing for major and minor determinants is just when the drug becomes needed in treatment. Testing to confirm a previous sensitivity to penicillin at a time when the medication is not required for the treatment of a specific condition is not recommended in most cases because of the possibility of developing sensitivity between the last testing and the next exposure.

Emergency allergic reactions

Triggers   **Most allergic emergencies concerning the dentist are drug-induced anaphylactic reactions.** The dentist must also be ready for reactions to anesthetics, vaccines, insect stings, foods, and injected dyes, and for transfusion reactions, aspirin sensitivities, hereditary angioedema, and cold-induced urticaria.

Manifestations   Anaphylactic reactions occur when a patient becomes overwhelmed by a sudden release of chemical mediators from mast cells. The onset is usually sudden, can be characterized by bronchospasm, wheezing, laryngeal edema, rash, or hives, and can cause a drop in blood pressure that can lead to life-threatening shock.

Emergency treatment of anaphylaxis

While the triggering agent of an acute allergic reaction is variable, the approach to handling the emergency is similar in most cases. The dentist's primary responsibility in an allergic emergency is to stabilize the patient until he or she can be transferred to an emergency facility or until assistance arrives. Whatever the degree of severity, all anaphylactic reactions must be evaluated quickly and carefully. Early treatment usually improves the prognosis and often decreases the severity of the reactions.

Airway and breathing

The patient's airway must be kept clear. Continual evaluation of the patient's respiratory and cardiovascular status is vital.

Recommended agents   **Injectable epinephrine 1:1,000 dilution** is the first-line drug in patients with bronchospasm and respiratory distress in whom there are no medical contraindications for such therapy. Dosage: 0.01 mg/kg body weight, not to exceed 0.3 cc. Can be repeated after 10 to 30 minutes, if required, and if the patient tolerated the previous dose well.

   A bronchodilator such as intravenous aminophylline should also be considered. In addition, **oxygen** by face mask or nasal prongs should be administered.

Other symptoms

Patients showing immediate hypersensitivity reactions of hives, swelling, bronchospasm, and anaphylactic shock should be stabilized as quickly as possible and, if indicated, transferred to the nearest emergency facility. **A list of emergency telephone numbers and the locations of nearby emergency rooms should be readily available in the dental office.** In severe cases, it may be necessary to begin an IV immediately to administer fluids and medications.

Recommended agents   Medications that are most helpful in anaphylactic emergencies include **antihistamines, bronchodilators,** and **corticosteroids**.

   Antihistamines should be injected intramuscularly at doses appropriate for the patient's body size. Injectable **diphenhydramine** or **hydroxyzine** can be used. The drugs are administered intravenously or by subcutaneous or intramuscular injection. Other antihistamines such as chlorpheneramine malate can be used at the discretion of the clinician.

Table 9.2 Emergency treatment of allergic reaction

Immediate allergic reaction

1. Maintain airway, give O_2 6 L/min by mask

2. Call for medical assistance

3. Administer 0.2–0.3 cc of 1:1,000 epinephrine subcutaneously

4. If indicated (condition worsens) administer 50 mg Benadryl IM or IV

5. If indicated (condition worsens) administer 125 mg Sol-u-Medrol IM or IV

6. If condition continues to deteriorate, repeat epinephrine administration 10 min after initial dose

Delayed reaction

Oral antihistamines may be sufficient treatment

Corticosteroids can be given either intramuscularly or intravenously. Unlike antihistamines and bronchodilators, which appear to have more immediate effects, corticosteroids usually do not begin to effect a clinical change for 8 to 12 hours after their administration.

Table 9.2 summarizes emergency treatment of anaphylaxis.

Summary

The dentist must stabilize the patient and act quickly and accurately until the patient can be transferred safely to an emergency facility or until assistance arrives. The dental practitioner should remain calm, evaluate the clinical problem quickly and accurately, and then initiate therapy.

Nonimmunologic drug reactions

Not all drug sensitivities have allergic or immunologic bases. Many drug reactions are not interactions between antigen and antibody. All persons are at risk to develop nonimmunologic drug reactions. Nonallergic drug reactions are no more likely in atopic than in nonatopic persons.

Some patients develop toxic side effects and unwanted reactions even when taking a drug as directed and within the therapeutic range. Examples of toxic side effects include drowsiness due to antihistamines, muscle tremor from terbutaline, stomach upset from aspirin or erythromycin, and hyperplasia of the gingiva from dilantin.

Causes of toxic side effects

Overdose   Patients who take a medication in dosages above the therapeutic range may develop toxic overdose, such as hemorrhage from the use of an anticoagulant.

Immunosuppressor drugs   Any patient is liable to develop an increased susceptibility to candidiasis, pneumocystis carinii pneumonia, or histoplasmosis when taking immunosuppressor drugs.

Drug interactions   When two drugs used concurrently have identical binding sites on the same cell they will compete, one will displace the other, and toxicity will result. Phenylbutazone displaces warfarin and results in bleeding. Phenylbutazone and salicylates displace tolbutamide and result in hypoglycemia.

Altered metabolism   In patients with hepatic or renal insufficiencies, toxicity might result from impaired metabolism or excretion of drugs that are metabolized in the liver and in the kidneys. Morphine is detoxified poorly by the cirrhotic patient. Streptomycin, digitalis, and potassium all accumulate during renal failure. When a patient is using digitalis and a diuretic is added, potassium loss may occur. As a result, the patient may develop an increased susceptibility to digitalis and become toxic. Toxicity can occur in asthmatic patients taking theophylline who develop cirrhosis of the liver, because theophylline clearance markedly decreases with the liver disorder.

Genetic defects   Sometimes genetic defects, such as inherited enzyme deficiency, surface as apparent drug sensitivities. Glucose-6-phosphate dehydrogenase deficiency can result in hemolytic anemia and hyperbilirubinemia after exposure to certain drugs such as antimalarials, sulfonamides, aspirin, and phenacetin.

Symptoms mimicking allergy

"Drug reaction" frequently creates the image of an atopic, wheezing, hives- and shock-prone person. This is not usually the case, although drug reactions sometimes mimic allergic reactions.

Rash   A maculopapular rash may develop from viral exanthem when ampicillin is used to treat infectious mononucleosis, certain viral infections, and other diseases. The virus can make the patient temporarily hypersensitive to enteric bacterial products or to the drug itself. Interaction between ampicillin and allopurinal can cause a rash due to hyperuricemia.

Histamine release   Morphine, codeine, atropine, pentamidine, polymyxin, meperidine, stilbamidine, and D-tubocurarine, which release histamine directly from cells without antigen-antibody reactions, can cause transient flushing, bronchospasm, urticaria, headache, and hypotension. Although it has not been clearly defined, a possible mechanism for some radiocontrast media reactions is the direct release of histamine from cells.

Aspirin intolerance is an idiosyncratic reaction, sometimes associated with asthma and nasal polyps or sensitivity to indomethacin and other non-steroidal anti-inflammatory drugs, naproxen, yellow dyes, or tartrazine. Symptoms in these patients, who are usually middle-aged nonallergic women, are similar to those of other idiosyncratic reactions and include wheezing and bronchospasm, transient flushing, and urticaria.

Drug withdrawal

Symptoms   Adverse withdrawal reactions and psychological drug reactions can arise when chronic drug treatment is stopped too abruptly. Symptoms associated with opiate withdrawal include nausea, anxiety, abdominal cramps, and hypertension. Withdrawal of diazepam and barbituates may result in irritability, delirium, seizures, and even death. Amphetamine withdrawal results in a "crash" and often a pattern of lassitude and sleep disturbance. "Rebound rhinitis" and obstruction may result when sympathomimetic nose drops use is abruptly halted.

Oral steroids   Oral steroid medication cutoff risks adrenal insufficiency. An oral surgery patient who has recently stopped taking oral steroids should be covered to prevent acute adrenal insufficiency. Use of steroids for 2 weeks within the previous 2 years usually requires supplemental steroid administration.

Further reading

de Weck, A.L. 1978. Drug reactions. pp. 413–439. *In* M. Samter (ed.) *Immunological Diseases.* 3rd ed. Boston: Little, Brown & Co.

Green, G.R., et al. 1977. Evaluation of penicillin hypersensitivity. *J. Allergy Clin. Immunol.* 60:339–345.

Ter, A.L. 1978. p. 514. *In* H. H. Fudenberg (ed.) *Basic and Clinical Immunology.* 2nd ed. Los Altos: Lange Publ. Co.

Van Arsdal, P.P. 1978. p. 1133. *In* E. Middleton, Jr. (ed.) *Allergy.* St. Louis: The C.V. Mosby Co.

CHAPTER 10

Adverse Microbiological Effects

Michael G. Newman, D.D.S.
Mahnaz Moussavi, D.D.S.

Antibiotics can temporarily and sometimes permanently alter the body's normal flora, thus rendering the patient more vulnerable to exogenous and endogenous infection. It is therefore prudent to prescribe antibiotics and antimicrobials conservatively, only when indicated and always with the most efficacious agent (see **Table 10.1**).

Development of bacterial resistance

The tendency toward development of bacterial resistance poses a serious ethical problem to the dentist. Resistance to some antibiotics can result when these drugs are used to treat a non-life-threatening orofacial infection or when they are used without being clearly indicated. **The danger is that the antibiotic may be ineffective if administered in the future for a truly serious infection. Thus, it is critical that these powerful drugs only be prescribed when absolutely indicated and for an appropriate duration.**

In general, any exposure to antibiotics tends to favor development of resistance within the bacterial flora. Resistance may be transferred from nonpathogenic to pathogenic species or it may be developed individually by specific bacteria.

The development of resistance to an antibiotic may involve a stable and persistent change in the genetic makeup of a particular bacterial species. The tendency toward development of resistance varies with the microorganism and with the drug. Group A *Streptococcus pyogenes*, for example, has not developed significant resistance to penicillin G over 35 years, whereas *Staphylococcus aureus* showed penicillin resistance soon after the drug was introduced.

Regional geographic patterns of bacterial resistance may also occur. In the near future regional standards of bacterial susceptibility may be required for efficacious prescription of antibiotics. Local hospital or dental school laboratories or national laboratories are good sources for further information.

Mechanisms through which resistance can arise:

1. Natural selection of strains showing resistance through random mutation, or
2. Movement of genetic material from a resistant strain to another microorganism, which then becomes resistant through transduction, transformation, or conjugation.

Superinfection

Infection with a species or strain of pathogenic microorganism (including viruses) or fungus different than that being treated can result from antibiotic use.

Depression of normal organisms   The bacteria and fungi that normally inhabit the skin and gastrointestinal, genitourinary, and respiratory tracts are depressed to varying degrees by antibacterial drugs. All antibiotics can produce a generalized depression of these nonpathogenic flora. The depression creates the potential for commensal pathogenic organisms resistant to the current treatment antibiotic to initiate a superinfection.

Symptoms   The gastrointestinal system is the most common site of superinfection following treatment of an odontogenic infection with oral antibiotics. Common symptoms include oral pain, xerostomia, glossitis, candidiasis, cheilosis, black hairy tongue, diarrhea, enteritis, colitis, and pruritus ani (see **Table 10.1**).

Candidiasis

Candidiasis is an overgrowth of a common oral commensal, the yeast *Candida albicans*. The disease is not common, occurring most often in the severely ill patient or as a side effect of antibiotic therapy. Antibiotic therapy with penicillin or a similar drug causes candidiasis by killing or depressing the normal flora with subsequent overgrowth of *Candida* organisms into the "microbiologic void." Candidiasis may occur as early as the fifth day of antibiotic therapy, but it more commonly begins after 10 to 14 days. Vaginal candidiasis occurs in a similar pattern and time period. Vaginal itching and burning are the primary symptoms (see chapter 19).

Treatment   When candidiasis is superficial and a result of antibiotic therapy, the agent of choice for its treatment is nystatin. The drug is given as a lozenge (Mycostatin Pastille®, 100,000 units) which is held in the mouth until it dissolves. Clotrimazole lozenges (Mycelex®, 10 mg) may also be used effectively. These drugs are used four to five times per day for 10 to 14 days. Deep-seated yeast or fungus infections do not normally occur as a complication of antibiotic therapy, but when they do occur because of other reasons they require other drugs and medical consultation.

Table 10.1   Symptoms of adverse microbiological effects

Effect	*Symptoms*
Superinfection	Oral pain
	Xerostomia
	Glossitis
	Candidiasis
	Cheilosis
	Black hairy tongue
	Diarrhea
	Enteritis
	Colitis
	Vaginitis
	Pruritus ani
Bacterial resistance	Failure of clinical response
	Deterioration of patient
	Possible resistance of future infections

The use of chlorhexidine gluconate 0.12% (Peridex®) is also used for superficial candidiasis, for example in cases of denture stomatitis (see chapter 15).

Antibiotic-associated colitis and diarrhea

Antibiotic use has been associated with diarrhea, ranging in severity from a mild self-limited problem to enterocolitis.[1] Diarrhea has been defined as five or more loose bowel movements per day. Antibiotic-associated diarrhea has been separated into three groups based on pathology present in the colon: pseudomembranous colitis, nonspecific colitis, and diarrhea without colitis.[2,4]

Finney[3] differentiated diarrheal enterocolitis following surgery of the gastrointestinal tract from the antibiotic-associated colitis not related to bowel surgery.

Etiology

Toxin-producing *Clostridium difficile* has been shown to be the most frequent etiologic agent of antibiotic-induced colitis.[5]

Antibiotic causes   Many antibiotic agents in both oral and parenteral forms have been

131

Table 10.2   Features of pseudomembranous colitis
(Patients reporting any of these symptoms should consult with a
physician trained in gastroenterology.)

- Watery diarrhea
- Bloody diarrhea in few cases, most commonly with ampicillin
- Diarrhea that persists for more than 48 hours
- Abdominal cramps
- Fever, elevated white blood cell count
- Possible late onset, several weeks after cessation of antibiotic therapy

---

implicated. The most commonly associated agents are lincomycin, clindamycin, and ampicillin, but other agents, including tetracyclines and cephalosporins, have been reported.[2]

Antibiotic-associated diarrhea does not appear to be dose-related. It is, however, age-related; risk increases with age.

Frequency   In relation to antibiotics, diarrhea has been shown to have a varied incidence in hospitalized patients. Diarrhea after clindamycin has been reported in from 6% to 21% of patients, with subsequent pseudomembranous colitis occurring in up to 10% of these patients.[6-10] Ampicillin has been associated with a 17% incidence of diarrhea and a 0.7% incidence of pseudomembranous colitis in one series.[6]

Symptoms

The patient can present with bloody diarrhea (most commonly with ampicillin), watery diarrhea, nausea, cramps, abdominal pain, and low-grade fever. The symptoms may start while the patient is on antibiotic therapy *or even up to 3 weeks after therapy is stopped*[2] (see **Table 10.2**).

Treatment

Most instances of pseudomembranous colitis resolve spontaneously, although consultation with the patient's physician is recommended because fluid loss can lead to electrolyte imbalance.

When the symptoms persist and are severe, the patient should be referred for endoscopic examination of the colon and stool assay for *C. difficile* toxin. Oral vancomycin is the antibiotic used to treat this colitis in severe cases. Cholestyramine resins are also used to bind the toxin. Occasionally, toxic megacolon will develop, which requires surgical intervention.[5]

Prophylaxis

The debate over whether to use yogurt or *Lactobacillus acidophilus* to make the bowel flora more "normal" as a prophylactic measure against diarrhea has not been resolved since Metchnikoff and Pasteur. A commercial preparation of *L. acidophilus*, Lactinex®, has been used prophylactically in some studies, but results are still unclear.

Contraception failure

Contemporary birth control pills have very low doses of estrogen to minimize their side effects. A portion of the bile excreted-estrogen is hydrolyzed by the gut flora and reabsorbed, creating an enterohepatic recirculation. Antibiotics such as tetracycline, penicillin, amoxicillin, and cephalosporins may alter the composition of the gut flora, thus preventing conversion of the estrogen metabolites back to an absorbable form. The result is a lowered plasma level of estrogen and a consequent increase in the chance for failure of contraception control. When the antibiotic is discontinued, the normal flora balance will recur, with eventual restoration of a normal estrogen balance. **The clinician who prescribes an antibiotic to a patient taking birth control pills should caution her to be aware of the possibility of breakthrough bleeding and decreased contraception control.**

Conclusions

Periodic review of drug package inserts and the current literature will keep the therapist adequately informed of constantly changing patterns of resistance. The most important contribution to the patient's health is prudent and conservative antibiotic prescription.

References

1. George, L., Sutter, V., and Finegold, S.M. 1977. Antimicrobial agent-induced diarrhea — a bacteria disease. *J. Infect. Dis.* 136:822.
2. George, L. 1982. Postoperative pseudomembranous enterocolitis. p. 286. *In* S. Wilson et al. (ed.) *Intra-abdominal infection.* New York: McGraw-Hill Book Co.
3. Finney, J.M.T. 1893. Gastro-enterostomy for cicatrizing ulcer of the pylorus. *In* Proceedings of the meeting of February 20, 1893. *Johns Hopkins Med. Bull.* 4:53–55.
4. Gorbach, S., and Bartlett, J. 1977. Pseudomembranous enterocolitis: a review of its diverse forms. *J. Infect. Dis.* 135 Suppl. S89.
5. George, L., Rolfe, R., and Finegold, S.M. 1980. Treatment and prevention of antimicrobial agent-

induced colitis and diarrhea. *Gastroenterology* 79:366.

6. Lusk, R., et al. 1977. Gastrointestinal side effect of clindamycin and ampicillin therapy. *J. Infect. Dis.* 135 Suppl. 111.

7. Swartzberg, T., Maresca, R., and Remington, J. 1977. Clinical study of gastrointestinal complications associated with clindamycin therapy. *J. Infect. Dis.* 135 Suppl. 99.

8. Gurwith, M., et al. 1977. Diarrhea associated with clindamycin and ampicillin therapy: preliminary results of a cooperative study. *J. Infect. Dis.* 135 Suppl. 104.

9. Neu, H., et al. 1977. Incidence of diarrhea and colitis associated with clindamycin therapy. *J. Infect. Dis.* 135 Suppl. 120.

10. Tedesco, F. 1977. Clindamycin and colitis: a review. *J. Infect. Dis.* 135 Suppl. 95.

PART 4

CLINICAL APPLICATION

CHAPTER 11

Antibiotics in Periodontal Therapy

Sebastian Ciancio, D.D.S.

Overview

The most common forms of periodontal disease — gingivitis and periodontitis — are caused by the presence of specific bacteria adjacent to or associated with periodontal structures. These bacteria, along with calculus and other local factors, are the principal components that perpetuate the disease process (see chapter 2). Therapy is focused on identifying, removing, and controlling these factors by a variety of mechanical and chemotherapeutic methods.

In many patients, systemic and local host factors influence the nature and severity of disease. The physiologic and psychologic status contribute to the extent and severity of the periodontal lesion and often influence the choice and response to therapy. Severe and/or acute periodontal and gingival infection often affect the general health status of the patient. In compromised individuals, periodontal infections can be life-threatening.

All periodontal diseases are not the same Gingivitis, defined as inflammation of the gingiva, can be further classified based on cause, pathogenesis, and host factors (see **Table 11.1**).

There are four major forms of periodontitis, comprising "related but distinct diseases that differ in etiology, natural history, progression and response to therapy"[1] (see **Table 2.2**). The natural history of the disease suggests that destruction of connective tissue attachment to the tooth is associated with periods of active destruction and relative quiesence. The periodontal tissues remain chronically inflamed histologically, but clinically the gingiva may or may not exhibit usual signs of inflammation.

Recognition and understanding of the causes and pathogenesis of these diseases is a prerequisite for establishing a rationale for antimicrobial and antibiotic therapy.

Limited use of antibiotics Debridement should *always* be tried before antibiotics in

Table 11.1   When to use systemic antibiotics*

Gingivitis	• Acute superficial infection associated with bacteremia and septicemia or associated with systemic disease
Acute necrotizing ulcerative gingivitis	• When severe and/or systemic symptoms are present
Periodontitis	• Localized juvenile
	• Early onset
	• Refractory
	• Acute, diffuse abscess
Periodontal surgical therapy implants	• Periodontal regenerative techniques
	• Postsurgical infection treatment and prophylaxis

*Topical chlorhexidine is always recommended concomitantly with systemic antibiotic treatment. Chlorhexidine may be continued for 2 to 3 days after cessation of antibiotics.

Table 11.2   Response of periodontium to antibiotics
Animal studies

Study	Results
Shaw et al. (1961)[13]	Antibiotics reduced periodontal syndrome in rice rat.
Stahl et al. (1962–1964)[14]	Antibiotics improved wound healing in animals but results were not long-lasting.
Wilderman (1963)[15]	Antibiotics did not improve wound healing in animals.
Shafer et al. (1964)[16]	Antibiotics improved wound healing in animals and less bone loss was seen after osseous recontouring.
Weiner et al. (1979)[17]	In induced periodontitis in animals, tetracyclines resulted in less alveolar bone resorption, less apical migration of junctional epithelium, and lowered levels of inflammatory cells in gingiva.
Heijl et al. (1982)[18]	Use of metronidazole was not superior to scaling, root planing, and tooth polishing in terms of plaque reduction and gingival health.
Toth et al. (1986)[19]	Minocycline inhibited bone loss in rice rats.
Chang et al. (1989)[20]	Minocycline stabilized collagen in rat gingiva.

periodontal therapy. In general, antibiotics are seldom necessary for treating most periodontal diseases. Debridement usually negates the need for antibiotics, especially in cases of minor acute necrotizing ulcerative gingivitis (ANUG) and localized periodontal abscess. Poor response to debridement or the presence of systemic manifestations of infection may indicate that host factors are contributing or that bacteria are within the periodontal tissue.

When to use antibiotics   Antibiotics can be valuable as treatment adjuncts in periodontal therapy when microorganisms occur in the connective tissue of diseased gingiva. Antibiotics are also somewhat successful in reducing plaque but they should *never* be prescribed for that purpose. As with other bacterial infections, the most effective agent against a periodontal disease is determined according to the dominant microorganisms in the infected area.

Microbiology   Although **Table 2.3** suggests that gram-positive bacteria are related to gingivitis, as the disease becomes more severe, the plaque progressively undergoes ecologic changes and gram-negative bacteria prevail. There is also an increase in anaerobic and motile bacteria as the gingival infection becomes more severe. In periodontitis, as the pocket deepens, the gram-negative capnophilic and anaerobic bacteria proliferate. For example, increased numbers of *Bacteroides gingivalis* and other *Bacteroides* sp. and spirochetes have been associated with deep periodontal pockets.[2] In juvenile periodontitis, recent studies strongly suggest that *Actinobacillus actinomycetemcomitans* are found in developing and established pockets and these organisms are etiologically related to the disease.[3] Some studies have suggested that in deep pockets bacteria may be found within gingival tissue.[4] Chapter 2 discusses the nature of the microbiota isolated from patients with periodontal diseases.

Gingivitis and plaque

Effectiveness of antibiotics

When antibiotics have been used topically or systemically to reduce or prevent plaque formation or gingivitis, the results have been favorable while the antibiotic was in use but the positive effects have not persisted after cessation of therapy.[3] Long-term use of therapeutic doses of antibiotics is contraindicated for many reasons, including the increased risk of side effects. The most likely side effects are development of resistant strains by natural selection and plasmid formation (see chapter 10).

Research with specific antibiotics   **Spiramycin, vancomycin, kanamycin, metronidazole,** and **erythromycin** have been tested for effectiveness as both preventive and therapeutic agents against gingivitis and plaque.[5,6] **Vancomycin** and **kanamycin** cannot be absorbed through the intestine, which limits their use in general medicine but enhances their potential for topical use in dentistry. In one study **kanamycin** was applied topically for 5 days to the teeth of mentally retarded children who had large amounts of plaque and severe gingivitis.[5] Supragingival plaque mass was reduced for 4 weeks, apparently due to the depression of plaque streptococci. This reduction was not significant, however, and because it occurred without mechanical oral hygiene, further investigation is needed.

Two studies showed some reduction of plaque and gingivitis with **kanamycin** and **metronidazole,** but not enough to warrant general use of the agents.[5,6]

The U.S. Food and Drug Administration prohibits use of **spiramycin** because of the associated high incidence of gastrointestinal problems. Effective mainly against gram-positive organisms, the drug reduces both gingivitis and plaque when administered systemically. Improvement has been reported in short-term studies of patients treated with spiramycin even when local therapy was not provided.[7,8]

Topical versus systemic   Antibiotics taken systemically can be advantageous in gingivitis and plaque treatment. Bacteriostatic and bacteriocidal levels of **penicillin, tetracycline, minocycline,** and **sulfonilamide** have been detected in saliva, and levels of **tetracycline, minocycline, doxycycline, metronidazole,** and **clindamycin** have been detected in gingival crevicular fluid after these agents were taken systemically. This places the antibiotics in intimate contact with both subgingival and supragingival plaque, focusing their activities where periodontal disease occurs.

The topical route of antibiotic administration may be less desirable because some antibiotics, notably penicillin, are more likely to cause hypersensitivity. Topical antibiotics can be absorbed through the oral mucosa causing systemic effects, including the development of resistant strains. In some cases plaque absorption and tooth adsorption can help reduce plaque. **Vancomycin, erythromycin, kanamycin, tetracycline,** and **bacitracin** have been tested topically with varying degrees of success.[7,9–12] Chapters 6 and 7 discuss topical antimicrobials in detail.

Periodontitis

When to use antibiotics   Antibiotics used systemically for the treatment of periodontal conditions must be carefully chosen, and patients must be frequently monitored. Antibiotics have been used as adjuncts to surgical therapy, to prevent the need for surgery in some cases, and to enhance the success of regenerative procedures.

In general, culture and susceptibility tests should be performed whenever an unusual or refractory infection is present. Topical chlorhexidine is recommended concomitantly with all systemic antibiotic treatment for at least 2 to 3 days after cessation of the antibiotic.

Table 11.1 lists clinical situations when antibiotics are commonly used. **Use of antibiotics in these situations is not automatic.** Each patient and their individual circumstances must be considered.

Table 11.3   Response of periodontium to antibiotics
Human studies

Study	Results
Winer et al. (1966)[21]	Spiramycin improved results of surgical and nonsurgical therapy.
Ariaudo (1969)[22]	Lincomycin reduced postoperative complications.
Dal Pra (1972)[23]	Penicillin reduced postoperative complications.
DeMarco et al. (1972)[24]	Clindamycin reduced postoperative necrosis but not postoperative complications.
Kidd et al. (1974)[25]	Phenoxymethyl penicillin reduced postoperative complications.
Scopp et al. (1977)[26]	Tetracycline did not reduce postoperative complications.
Slots et al. (1979)[27]	Suggested tetracyclines may be useful adjuncts to periodontal therapy.
Pendrill et al. (1980)[28]	Penicillin reduced postoperative pain following periodontal surgery.
Ciancio et al. (1980)[29]	Minocycline concentrated in crevicular fluid, reduced crevicular bacteria, and improved gingival health.
Loesche et al. (1981)[5]	Metronidazole reduced crevicular bacteria and improved periodontal health.
Ciancio et al. (1982)[30]	Minocycline improved gingival health. Suggested minocycline may be useful adjunct to mechanical therapy.
Appleman et al. (1982)[31]	Cephalexin reduced the incidence of polymicrobic bacteremia in periodontal surgery but had no significant effect on wound healing.
Golub et al. (1984)[32]	Minocycline inhibits tissue collagenolytic activity by a mechanism not dependent on the drug's antibacterial properties.
Schmidt et al. (1988)[33]	No significant effects of metronidazole on alveolar bone regeneration.

Antibiotic selection   The agent chosen to treat periodontitis should be one that will:

1. Travel readily to the infection site and concentrate in therapeutic levels in the crevicular fluid and gingival tissue
2. Have minimal host and microbial side effects
3. Have a positive benefit-to-risk ratio

Tables **11.2** and **11.3** summarize results obtained in studies on animals and humans where antibiotics were used as adjuncts in periodontitis therapy.

Penicillin

Penicillin is contraindicated topically because this route of administration readily results in hypersensitivity reactions, compromising its value as a life-saving antibiotic.

Systemic administration of penicillin, particularly broad-spectrum agents such as amoxicillin, is of value as initial therapy for both periapical and periodontal abscess in conjunction with draining when possible and for acute necrotizing ulcerative gingivitis (ANUG) when severe pain, fever, or lymphodenopathy is associated with this condition.

Amoxicillin may be useful alone or in combination with clavulanic acid (Augmentin®) and metronidazole (see below) in the management of patients with refractory or early-onset forms of periodontitis. In some studies, patients not responsive to tetracyclines, clindamycin, or metronidazole alone have improved when the drugs were prescribed using susceptibility data.[34,35]

Augmentin

Augmentin consists of amoxicillin and clavulanic acid (see chapter 5). Although the pathogens affected by Augmentin have not been fully identified, they are known to include both gram-positive and gram-negative bacteria.

Tetracyclines

The tetracyclines concentrate in gingival crevicular fluid at levels five to seven times those in serum.[36,37] Many of the microorganisms found in deep periodontal pockets are sensitive to the drug.

Unlike other antibiotics (such as penicillin), tetracycline is particularly effective against *A. actinomycetemcomitans*, which is etiologically associated with juvenile periodontitis. Also in contrast with other antibiotics, including metronidazole, tetracyclines may protect collagen and thereby strengthen host resistance by inhibiting the production of endogenous collagenase.

Despite generally positive attributes of tetracycline, a number of studies have indicated that it should not replace conventional therapy. Tetracyclines appear to be effective in the treatment of many patients with juvenile periodontitis and rapidly advancing periodontitis, and in some cases of refractory periodontitis. Kornman et al.[38] evaluated the effects of tetracycline after administration for up to 7 years in 20 patients who were refractory to conventional periodontal treatment. Although many of the patients improved, the organisms associated with periodontal disease returned when treatment was discontinued. High levels of tetracycline-resistant organisms were seen in four of the ten patients.

The major side effects of tetracyclines include gastrointestinal disturbances, photosensitivity, kidney and liver dysfunction, discoloration of mucosa and tooth extraction sockets, tooth discoloration in children when given during the time of tooth crown formation, and superinfection with *Candida albicans*, particularly in debilitated patients.

Further research is needed before tetracycline can be recommended for adult patients who have not responded to periodontal treatment with scaling and root planing.

Minocycline   A semisynthetic tetracycline that is effective against a similarly broad spectrum of microorganisms. It has been reported that minocycline suppressed spirochetes and motile rods as effectively as scaling and root planing in patients with adult periodontitis, with the suppression being evident for up to 3 months after therapy.[29,30] Compared with other tetracyclines, which generally require administration four times a day, minocycline can be given twice a day. Also, it is associated with less renal toxicity and phototoxicity. However, minocycline may cause reversible vertigo.

Doxycycline   Has the same spectrum of activity as minocycline and might be equally effective. Because it can be given once daily, doxycycline favors compliance.

In mixtures   Because tetracyclines are purported to cause fungal overgrowth in mucous membranes of the gastrointestinal tract and vagina, they are available for prescription in combinations with antifungal agents (see chapter 19). However, there has been no convincing evidence in the medical-dental literature that such mixtures result in decreased fungal infections, although there may be a rational base for their use in patients who are diabetic, debilitated, or receiving adrenal corticosteroids (see chapter 18).

Metronidazole

Metronidazole is highly effective against the anaerobic bacteria associated with periodontal disease. Recent studies have suggested that, when combined with amoxicillin or Augmentin, metronidazole may be of value in managing some patients with juvenile and refractory periodontitis.[34,35]

Levels of metronidazole in crevicular fluid are slightly higher than those found in serum, resulting in concentrations that are lethal to many plaque bacteria.

In some trials, metronidazole has demonstrated a beneficial effect on periodontitis when used in conjunction with good oral hygiene and/or subgingival debridement.[39] As with other antibiotics, the effects of metronidazole were reduced when used alone.

The major side effects of metronidazole include metallic taste sensations, headache, vertigo, peripheral neuritis, and gastrointestinal disturbances, particularly when combined with alcohol. The interaction with alcohol is so severe that **use of alcohol should be prohibited when taking metronidazole.**

Clindamycin

Clindamycin is effective against the bacteria associated with periodontal disease.[40] It has shown efficacy in patients with periodontitis who were refractory to tetracycline or metronidazole therapy.[40] However, because the use of this antibiotic has been associated with pseudomembraneous colitis more often than other antibiotics, its use is limited and caution is advised.

Mode of delivery

Periodontal dressings

Some authors have claimed improved wound healing when antibiotics were applied in periodontal dressings, but the main advantage appears to be alleviation of the bad taste or odor beneath the dressings, which are sometimes observed after periodontal surgery. This limited value does not warrant use of antibiotics in dressings, especially because they are being applied to cut surfaces, which increases the probability of systemic absorption. Resistant strains can develop from the resultant exposure of body flora to low doses of antibiotics.

Crevicular placement/slow-release devices

Another route of administration involves placement of medication in the gingival crevice. Because periodontal disease is often characterized by many microulcerations, the crevicular epithelium is usually not intact. Therefore, crevicular placement of an agent may be more closely related to subcutaneous than to topical administration.

So far, chlorhexidine, tetracycline, and metronidazole have been investigated in slow-release devices. Most studies of local delivery have been done with tetracycline-loaded fibers.[41-44] When packed into gingival crevices or pockets, these fibers slowly release low doses of tetracycline over a period of 10 days, after which they are removed. Clinical trials to date have indicated that the use of these fibers shows promise as an adjunct to conventional therapeutic methods in the treatment of some forms of periodontal disease.

Application of antimicrobial agents to the subgingival area by means of slow-release devices appears to have great promise in altering the microbiota. In addition, investigations are currently under way to evaluate slow-release devices that are absorbable and therefore do not require removal. Further studies are needed to determine the dosage, duration, and efficacy of local drug delivery systems.

Irrigation

The use of chemical agents in irrigation devices is of interest because these devices can deliver aqueous solutions farther into the crevice or pocket than can rinsing. A recent study showed that a pulsated irrigation directed at the orifice of a pocket can penetrate to approximately half the depth of the pocket.[44,45] Additional studies have shown that when irrigation tips are placed 2 to 3 mm into a periodontal pocket, solutions can be delivered 6 to 9 mm.[46] These studies have produced enough data to establish safety and feasibility of irrigation with powered devices as a potential therapeutic modality. Although studies have demonstrated the efficacy of irrigation in treating gingivitis, definitive studies are not available relative to their role in the treatment of periodontitis.

Various medications have been evaluated as irrigants, including chlorhexidine, metronidazole, stannous fluoride, quaternary ammonium agents, sanguinarine, iodine, and essential oils. Most of these studies have been carried out for short time periods and have shown interesting reductions in gingivitis but no significant effects on periodontitis.

Use of various agents has shown that short-term irrigation (1 to 2 days) has resulted in a reduction of *Bacteroides* and spirochetes for 5 to 7 days.[47-49] When irrigation has been preceded by root planing, several studies have shown little improvement from irrigation, whereas others have suggested some benefit.[50-54] Although irrigation has resulted in small pocket reduction of 1 mm or less, root planing alone has been far more effective. A similar finding has been reported for bleeding on probing.

A recent study by Ciancio and coworkers[55] evaluated supragingival irrigation using Listerine® in a Water Pik®. Sixty-six adults were examined in a double-blind study to determine the effect of an antimicrobial agent delivered by an oral irrigating device. Each subject received a randomized half-mouth dental prophylaxis. The results of this study showed that an antimicrobial product delivered by an oral irrigating device could result in significant reductions in plaque, bacterial cell counts, and gingival bleeding and may therefore be an effective adjunct to normal oral hygiene.

The only 6-month irrigation study reported to date was one in which irrigation using a Water Pik with a chemical agent (0.06% chlorhexidine diluted, Peridex®) was compared to irrigation with water, rinsing with 0.12% chlorhexidine, or normal oral hygiene.[56] The results of this study conducted in over 160 patients showed the following in the reduction of gingivitis:

1. Irrigation with 0.06% chlorhexidine was more effective than irrigation with water, rinsing with 0.12% chlorhexidine, or normal oral hygiene.
2. Irrigation with water was equal to rinsing with 0.12% chlorhexidine and better than normal oral hygiene.
3. Bacterial reductions were better with chlorhexidine than with water.

Oral irrigation with chemical agents as an adjunct to therapy for gingivitis may be of value in the treatment of gingivitis and deserves further study as an adjunct to the treatment of periodontitis. *At the present time irrigation is not recommended in patients where transient bacteremia may be life threatening* (see chapter 17) even though some studies do not report an increase in bacteremias following irrigation.[57]

References

1. American Academy of Periodontology. 1989. *World Workshop in Clinical Periodontics*. Chicago: American Academy of Periodontology, pp. 1–23.

2. Slots, J. 1982. Importance of black-pigmented *Bacteroides* in human periodontal disease. p. 27. *In* R. Genco and S. Mergenhagen (eds.) *Host-parasite Interactions in Periodontal Disease*. Washington, D.C.: American Society for Microbiology.

3. Mandell, R.L., and Socransky, S.S. 1981. A selective medium for *Actinobacillus actinomycetemcomitans* and the incidence of the organism in juvenile periodontitis. *J. Periodontol.* 52:593.

4. Saglie, R., Newman, M.G., Carranza, F.A., Jr., and Pattison, G.L. 1982. Bacterial invasion of gingiva in advanced periodontitis in humans. *J. Periodontol.* 53:217.

5. Loesche, W.J., Syed, S.A., Morrison, E.C., Laughon, B., and Grassman, N.S. 1981. Treatment of periodontal infections due to anaerobic bacteria with short-term treatment with metronidazole. Case reports of five patients. *J. Clin. Periodontol.* 8:29.

6. Löe, H., Theilade, E., Jensen, S.G., and Schiott, C.R. 1967. Experimental gingivitis in man. III. The influence of antibiotics on gingival plaque development. *J. Periodont. Res.* 2:282–289.

7. Johnson, R.H., and Rozanis, J. 1979. A review of chemotherapeutic plaque control. *Oral Surg.* 47:136–141.

8. Mills, W.H., Thompson, G.W., and Beagrie, G.S. 1976. Double blind clinical evaluation of spiramycin and erythromycin in control of periodontal disease. *J. Dent. Res.* Vol. 55 (B), Abstr. no. 806.

9. Ciancio, S.G., and Bourgault, P. 1980. *Clinical Pharmacology for Dental Professionals*. New York: McGraw-Hill Book Co.

10. Hollander, L., and Hardy, S.M. 1950. The use of aureomycin ointment in dermatology. *Am. Prac. Digest Treat.* 1:54–57.

11. Jensen, S.G., Löe, H., Schiott, C.R., and Theilade, E. 1968. Experimental gingivitis in man. IV. Vancomycin induced changes in bacterial plaque composition as related to development of gingival inflammation. *J. Periodont. Res.* 3:284–293.

12. Loesche, W.J., and Nafe, D. 1973. Reduction of supragingival plaque accumulation in institutionalized Down's syndrome patients by periodic treatment with topical kanamycin. *Arch. Oral Biol.* 18:1131–1143.

13. Shaw, J.H., Griffiths, A., and Auskaps, T. 1961. The influence of antibiotics on the periodontal syndrome in the rice rat. *J. Dent. Res.* 40:511.

14. Stahl, S. 1962. The influence of antibiotics on the healing of gingival wounds in rats. *J. Periodontol.* 33:261.

15. Wilderman, M.N. 1963. Repair after a periosteal retention procedure. *J. Periodontol.* 34:487.

16. Shafer, T.J., Collings, C.K., Bishop, J.G., and Dorman, H.L. 1964. The effect of antibiotics on healing following osseous recontouring in dogs. *Periodontics* 3:243.

17. Weiner, G.S., DeMarco, T.J., Bissada, N.F. 1979. Long-term effects of systemic tetracycline administration on the severity of induced periodontics in the rat. *J. Periodontol.* 50:619.

18. Heijl, L., and Lindhe, J. 1982. The effect of metronidazole on established gingivitis and plaque in beagle dogs. *J. Periodontol.* 53:180.

19. Toth, A., Beck, F.M., Beck, E.X., Flaxman, N., and Rosen, S. 1986. Effect of antimicrobial agents on root surface caries, alveolar bone loss, and microflora in rice rats. *J. Dent. Res.* 65(5):695–697.

20. Chang, K.M., Ramamurthy, N.S., and Golub, L.M. 1989. Minocycline (MIN) inhibits matrix-degrading enzymes in rat gingiva. *J. Dent. Res.* 68:198 (Abstr. no. 130).

21. Winer, R.A., Cohen, M.M., and Chauncey, H.H. 1966. Antibiotic therapy in periodontal disease. *J. Oral Ther. Pharm.* 2:404.

22. Ariaudo, A.A. 1969. Efficacy of antibiotics in periodontal surgery. *J. Periodontol.* 40:150.

23. Dal Pra, D.J. 1972. A clinical evaluation of the benefits of a course of oral penicillin following periodontal surgery. *Aust. Dent. J.* 17:219.

24. DeMarco, T.J., and Kluth, E.V. 1972. The use of cleocin in post-surgical periodontal patients. *J. Periodontol.* 43:381.

25. Kidd, E.A.M., and Wade, A.B. 1974. Penicillin control of swelling and pain after periodontal osseous surgery. *J. Clin. Periodontol.* 1:52–57.

26. Scopp, I.W., Fletcher, P.D., Wyman, B.S., Epstein, S.R., and Fine, A. 1977. Tetracyclines: double blind clinical study to evaluate the effectiveness in periodontal surgery. *J. Periodontol.* 48:484.

27. Slots, J., Mashimo, P., Levine, M.J., and Genco, R.J. 1979. Periodontal therapy in humans. I. *J. Periodontol.* 50:495.

28. Pendrill, K., and Reddy, J. 1980. The use of prophylactic penicillin in periodontal surgery. *J. Periodontol.* 51:44–48.

29. Ciancio, S.G., Mather, M.L., and McMullen, J.A. 1980. An evaluation of minocycline in patients with periodontal disease. *J. Periodontol.* 51:530–534.

30. Ciancio, S.G., Slots, J., Reynolds, H., Zambon, J., and McKenna, J. 1982. The effect of short-term administration of minocycline HC1 on gingival inflammation and subgingival microflora. *J. Periodontol.* 53:557–561.

31. Appleman, M.D., Sutter, V.L., and Sims, T.N. 1982. Value of antibiotic prophylaxis in periodontal surgery. *J. Periodontol.* 53:319.

32. Golub, L.M., et al. 1984. Tetracyclines inhibit tissue collagenolytic enzyme activity: a new concept in the treatment of periodontal disease. *J. Dent. Res.* 63: Abstr. no. 869:267.

33. Schmidt, E.F., Webber, R.L., Ruttimann, U.E., and Loesche, W. 1988. Effect of periodontal therapy on alveolar bone as measured by subtraction radiography. *J. Periodontol.* 59:633–638.

34. Newman, M.G., Kornman, K.S., et al. 1989. Treatment of refractory periodontitis with Augmentin. *J. Dent. Res.* (Spec. Iss.) Abstr. no. 404.

35. Kornman, K.S., and Newman, M.G. 1989. Treatment of refractory periodontitis with metronidazole plus amoxicillin and Augmentin. *J. Dent. Res.* (Spec. Iss.) Abstr. no. 403.

36. Ciancio, S.G., Mather, M.L., and McMullen, J.A. 1980. An evaluation of minocycline in patients with periodontal disease. *J. Periodontol.* 51:530–534.

37. Gordon, J.M., Walker, C.B., Murphy, J.C., Goodson, J.M., and Socransky, S.S. 1981. Tetracycline: levels achievable in gingival crevice fluid and in vitro effect on subgingival organisms. Part. I. *J. Periodontol.* 52:609.

38. Kornman, K.S., and Robertson, P.B. 1985. Clinical and microbiological evaluation of therapy for juvenile periodontitis. *J. Periodontol.* 56:443.

39. Loesche, W.J., Syed, S.A., Morrison, E.C., et al. 1984. Metronidazole in periodontitis. I. Clinical and bacteriological results after 15 to 30 weeks. *J. Periodontol.* 55:325.

40. Tyler, K., Walker, C., Gordon, J., Pappas, J., and Cohen, S. 1985. Evaluation of clindamycin in adult refractory periodontitis: antimicrobial susceptibilities. *J. Dent. Res.* 64 (Spec. Iss.): Abstr. no. 1667.

41. Goodson, J.M., Haffajee, A., and Socransky, S.S. 1979. Periodontal therapy by local delivery of tetracycline. *J. Clin. Periodontol.* 6:83–92.

42. Goodson, J.M., Holborrow, D., Dunn, R.L., Hogan, P., and Dunham, S. 1983. Monolithic tetracycline-containing fibers of controlled delivery to periodontal pockets. *J. Periodontol.* 54:575.

43. Soskolne, A., Golumb, G., Friedman, M., and Sela, M.N. 1983. New sustained release dosage form of chlorhexidine for dental use. II. Use in periodontal therapy. *J. Periodont. Res.* 18:33.

44. Addy, M., Hassan, H., Moran, J., Wade, W., and Newcombe, R. 1988. Use of antimicrobial containing acrylic strips in the treatment of chronic periodontal disease. A three month follow-up study. *J. Periodontol.* 59:557.

45. Eakle, W.S., Ford, C., and Boyd, R. 1986. Depth of penetration in periodontal pockets with oral irrigation. *J. Clin. Periodontol.* 13:39.

46. Hollander, R., Boyd, R.L., and Eakle, W. 1989. Comparison of canula versus standard tip for oral irrigation. *J. Dent. Res.* 68:410 (Abstr. no. 1829).

47. Larner, J., Robinson, P., and Lautenschlager, E. 1989. Penetrability of periodontal pockets with various subgingival tip designs. *J. Dent. Res.* 68:410 (Abstr. no. 1830).

48. Westling, M., and Tynelius-Bratthal, G. 1984. Microbial and clinical short-term effects of repeated intracrevicular chlorhexidine rinsings. *J. Periodont. Res.* 19:202.

49. Baer, P.N., Limbardi, R.J., and Cox, D.S. 1986. Effect of H_2O_2 solution delivered to the base of

periodontal pocket on pigmented *Bacteroides. J. Dent. Res.* 65:182 (Abstr. no. 1110).

50. Schmid, E., Kornman, K., and Tinanoff, N. 1985. Changes of subgingival colony forming units and black-pigmented *Bacteroides* after a single irrigation of periodontal pockets with 1.64% SnF$_2$. *J. Periodontol.* 56:330.

51. Wennstrom, J., Dahlen, G., Grondahl, K., and Heijl, L. 1987. Periodic subgingival antimicrobial irrigation of pockets. II. Microbiologic and radiographic observation. *J. Clin. Periodontol.* 14:573.

52. Macauley, W.J., and Newman, H.N. 1986. The effect on the composition of subgingival plaque of a simplified oral hygiene system including pulsating jet subgingival irrigation. *J. Periodont. Res.* 21:375.

53. MacAlpine, R., Magnusson, I., Kiger, R., et al. 1985. Antimicrobial irrigation of deep pockets to supplement oral hygiene instruction and root debridement. I. Bi-weekly irrigation. *J. Clin. Periodontol.* 12:568.

54. Krust, K., Drisko, C., Gross, K., Overman, P., and Tira, D. 1989. A comparison of subgingival irrigation with chlorhexidine and stannous fluoride. *J. Dent. Res.* 68: Abstr. no. 1831.

55. Ciancio, S.G., Mather, M.L., Zambon, J.J., and Reynolds, H.S. 1989. Effect of a chemotherapeutic agent delivered by an oral irrigation device on plaque, gingivitis, and subgingival microflora. *J. Periodontol.* 6(6):310.

56. Flemmig, T.F., Newman, M.G., Doherty, F.M., Grossman, E., Meckle, A.H., and Bakdash, B. 1990. Supragingival irrigation with 0.06% chlorhexidine in naturally occurring gingivitis. I. 6 month clinical observations. *J. Periodontol.* 61:112.

57. Waki, M., et al. 1990. Effects of subgingival irrigation on bacteremia following scaling and root planing. *J. Periodontol.* 61:405–411.

Further reading

Ciancio, S.G. 1976. Tetracycline and periodontal therapy. *J. Periodontol.* 47:155–159.

Ciancio, S.G., and Bourgault, P.C. 1980. *Clinical Pharmacology for Dental Professionals.* New York: McGraw-Hill Book Co., Inc.

Johnson, R.H., and Rozanis, J. 1979. A review of chemotherapeutic plaque control. *Oral Surg.* 47:136–141.

Loesche, W.J. 1976. Chemotherapy of dental plaque infections. *Oral Sci. Rev.* 9:65–107.

Parsons, J.C. 1974. Chemotherapy of dental plaque — a review. *J. Periodontol.* 45:177.

CHAPTER 12

Antibiotics in Endodontic Therapy

J. Craig Baumgartner, D.D.S., Ph.D.

Infections of endodontic origin

Since 1890, when Miller[1] first observed microorganisms associated with inflamed pulpal tissue, microorganisms have been implicated in infections of endodontic origin. This relationship was proven in 1965 when Kakehashi et al.[2] demonstrated that pulpal necrosis and the development of periapical inflammatory lesions only occur in conventional rats, not in germ-free rats, after exposure of the dental pulp to the oral cavity.

Pathways of endodontic infection

Pulpal exposure　The most common route that microorganisms take to reach the dental pulp is through a carious pulpal exposure in the crown of the tooth. Microorganisms may also reach the pulp via a pulpal exposure caused either by a traumatic injury or by an operative procedure.

Dentinal tubules　Microbes may reach the dental pulp through dentinal tubules exposed by enamel lamellae, dentinal tubules exposed by dental procedures, or from pressure on dentinal tubules produced by impression materials or restorative materials.

Lateral or furcation canals　Lateral or furcation canals exposed either by disease or dental treatment may also be portals of entry for microorganisms to the root canal system of a tooth. Deep periodontal infections expose these canals to large numbers of bacteria. Teeth adjacent to periodontal lesions may have periodontal bacteria deep within the dentinal tubules.

Other　There may be direct extension of an infection from an adjacent tooth or an anachoretic transport of microorganisms through the blood to an area of pulpal inflammation.[3]

Reservoir of infection

Once the pulpal tissue becomes necrotic and loses its blood supply, the root canal system becomes a reservoir for microorganisms and their by-products. Because of the lack of circulation within the necrotic pulp, the root canal is insulated from the normal host defense mechanisms of the body.

Microflora in infections of endodontic origin

Ecosystem   The microbial ecosystem in a root canal system is very complex and not fully understood. The selection of the microflora in an infected root canal system from hundreds of known microbial inhabitants of the oral cavity is determined by a variety of factors, including nutritional supply, oxidation-reduction potential, and microbial interactions.

Obligate anaerobes   With the development of anaerobic culturing methods, the predominance of obligate anaerobic bacteria was established (see **Table 12.1**). In addition, it has been well documented that infected root canals are usually polymicrobial in nature with several predominant anaerobic microorganisms.

Table 12.1   Isolates from infections of endodontic origin

| Source of sample | Total samples | Number of samples | | |
		with anaerobes	with anaerobes exclusively	with facultatives exclusively
Intact necrotic root canal systems[4]	19	18 (95%)	13 (67%)	2 (10%)
Intact necrotic root canal systems[5]	55	55 (100%)	18 (33%)	0 (0%)
Apical 5 mm of exposed root canal system[6]	10	10 (100%)	2 (20%)	0 (0%)
Orofacial odontogenic infection[7]	31	29 (95%)	13 (42%)	Not determined
Abscessed teeth in children[8]	12	12 (100%)	8 (67%)	0 (0%)
Abscesses of endodontic origin[9]	10	9 (90%)	6 (60%)	1 (10%)

Black-pigmented **Bacteroides**   Before 1976 there were no studies that could establish a correlation between the presence of a specific microorganism isolated from a root canal to clinical signs or symptoms. In 1976, Sundqvist[4] isolated anaerobic black-pigmented *Bacteroides* sp. from seven patients with acute pain. A study by Griffee et al.[10] partially supported the work of Sundqvist. Griffee et al. found that the presence of black-pigmented *Bacteroides* sp. in an infected root canal was related to pain, foul odor, and the presence of a sinus tract. Haapasalo et al.[11] isolated black-pigmented *Bacteroides* sp. from 54% of symptomatic patients and 44% of non-symptomatic patients. However, *Bacteroides endodontalis*, and *Bacteroides gingivalis* were only isolated from symptomatic teeth, whereas other strains of black-pigmented *Bacteroides* sp. were found in both symptomatic and asymptomatic teeth. In a more recent study, Sundqvist et al.[12] cultured black-pigmented *Bacteroides* sp. from 22 root canals of 72 teeth. Fourteen of the strains were *Bacteroides intermedius* and five strains were *B. endodontalis*. Sixteen of the 22 root canals (73%) infected with black-pigmented *Bacteroides* sp. were associated with apical abscesses and purulent drainage from the infected root canal. In a study designed to detect the presence of black-pigmented *Bacteroides* in odontogenic abscesses, Van Winkelhoff et al.[13] found that 26 of 28 (93%) samples of pus contained one or more species of black-pigmented *Bacteroides*.

Polymicrobial   Other strains of anaerobic microorganisms often isolated from infections of endodontic origin in addition to black-pigmented *Bacteroides* sp. include: *Peptostreptococcus* sp., *Eubacterium* sp., *Fusobacterium* sp., *Actinomyces* sp., *Veillonella* sp., *Propionibacterium* sp., and *Lactobacillus* (anaerobic) sp.[6,12] Microorganisms inhabiting an infected root canal are mostly anaerobic, but facultative microorganisms may occur in large numbers. Facultative anaerobes commonly isolated include: *Streptococcus (Enterococcus)* sp., *Lactobacillus* (aerobic) sp., and *Staphylococcus* sp. Although the above microorganisms have been associated with infections of endodontic origin, no single microbe or group of microbes has been proven to be more pathogenic than others. **From a clinical viewpoint, it is still best to consider all infections of endodontic origin as being polymicrobial and treat them accordingly.**

Periapical pathoses   Once the dental pulp becomes necrotic, microbial infection of the root canal system may contribute to a localized periapical inflammatory lesion, an abscess, or a diffuse cellulitis. The growth of microorganisms within the root canal system and subsequent irritation of the periapical tissue by their by-products will continue indefinitely or until the source of the irritation is removed. On occasion, bacteria overcome the host defenses and invade the periapical tissues. When this occurs the inhabitants of infected root canal systems can be cultured from the aspirates of abscesses of endodontic origin.[7-9,13] However, even without direct invasion, bacteria produce an enormous quantity of products that diffuse into the periapical tissues via apical and lateral canals, which provoke both specific and non-specific inflammatory reactions. The inflammatory response may give rise to both protective and immunopathogenic effects. The developing periapical inflammatory reaction to the irritants may be destructive to surrounding tissue and contribute to adverse signs and symptoms. Serious infections may develop, depending on the pathogenicity of the microorganisms involved and the resistance of the host.

Table 12.2 Treatment of infections of endodontic origin

Clinical findings	*Treatment approach*
• Uncomplicated endodontic lesion 　No compromised host resistance 　Pain resolves with drainage through root 　　canal 　No swelling	• Debridement of root canal system
• Soft tissue swelling of endodontic origin 　Well localized swelling 　No systemic signs such as: fever, 　　malaise, cellulitis	• Debridement of root canal system 　Soft tissue incisions and drainage
• Endodontic lesion confined to bone 　No soft tissue swelling 　Exquisite pain 　No drainage through root canal	• Trephination of bone to relieve pressure 　and speed healing
• Complicated endodontic lesion 　Compromised host response *or* 　Evidence of systemic involvement or 　　spread of infection such as: fever, 　　malaise, cellulitis	• Debridement of root canal system and 　systemic antibiotics (see **Table 12.3**)

Treatment of infections of endodontic origin (see **Table 12.2**)

Debridement and drainage

Root canal system　The key to successful management of infections of endodontic origin is chemomechanical **debridement** of the infected root canal system and **drainage** from both soft and hard tissues. The root canal system of the infected tooth should be allowed to drain and should be aseptically debrided to near its radiographic apex. It is important that debridement of the root canal be accomplished aseptically using a disinfected rubber dam and with sterile instruments to prevent further microbial contamination. The maintenance of a patent apical foramen with a small endodontic instrument (e.g., no. 15) will act as a vent for drainage from the periapical tissues through the root canal. The objectives for treatment of infections of endodontic origin are *(1)* removal of the pathogenic microorganisms, their by-products, and pulpal debris from the infected root canal system that caused the periapical pathosis, and *(2)* establishment of favorable conditions for the lesion to resolve. Because the microorganisms are found in tubules and in parts of the canal system not reached by endodontic instruments, an irrigating solution with antimicrobial and tissue dissolution properties, such as sodium hypochlorite, should be used. After drainage and debridement, the root canal system should be sealed. Either a sterile cotton pellet or a cotton pellet with a drop of an antimicrobial such as formocresol, cresatin, or camphorated parachlorophenol should be sealed into the pulp chamber with a temporary restoration until the final root canal filling is placed. The root canal should *not* be left open to contamination by the oral microflora.

Soft tissue incision and drainage   Soft tissue swelling of endodontic origin should be incised and drained concurrently with chemomechanical debridement of the root canal system. In most cases a rubber drain placed in the incision for 24 hours will allow for adequate drainage. Drainage allows the accumulated irritants and inflammatory mediators to be decreased to a level where a healthy host can initiate healing. In a healthy host, culture of such lesions and systemic antibiotics are usually unnecessary unless there is a delay in healing or later signs of spread of the infection.

Trephination   On occasion a patient will present with exquisite pain when it is not possible to obtain drainage through the root canal and no soft tissue swelling is present. With time the inflammatory mediators and pus will follow the pathway of least resistance and eventually perforate the cortical plate and elevate the periosteum. However, before destruction of the cortical plate, the lesion may not be evident radiographically, the restraint of fluids may cause the pressure to become extreme, and drainage through the root canal may be inadequate. Consideration should be given to the use of trephination, direct surgical penetration through the bone to the periapical lesion, which usually provides the patient with immediate relief. Postoperative care in such cases should include systemic antibiotics for 7 to 10 days (see **Table 12.3**).

Patients requiring prophylactic antibiotic coverage

Although the incidence of bacteremia is low, studies using aerobic and anaerobic culturing have demonstrated that a transient bacteremia can result from extrusion of microorganisms beyond the apex of a root as a result of over-instrumentation of a root canal.[14,15] Medically compromised patients at increased risk of infection must receive prophylactic antibiotics that follow the recommendations of the American Heart Association or an alternate regimen determined in consultation with the patient's physician.[16,17] Patients requiring prophylactic antibiotic treatment include those with rheumatic heart disease, congenital heart disease, heart murmurs, systemic-pulmonary shunts, mitral valve prolapse with insufficiency, uncontrolled diabetes, immunosuppressed or immunologically deficient patients, and patients with prosthetic joints or other types of implants.

Patients *not* requiring antibiotics

Healthy patients who present with a localized, fluctuant, intraoral swelling of endodontic origin do *not* require antibiotics. Likewise, healthy patients with a symptomatic pulpitis, symptomatic apical periodontitis, or a draining sinus tract do *not* require antibiotics. Debridement of the root canal system that is the reservoir of the infection and drainage of both soft and hard tissues as discussed above is the treatment of choice. Antibiotics should not be substituted for root canal debridement and adequate drainage of soft and hard tissues.

Patients requiring antibiotics to treat infection

Antibiotic therapy is indicated when there is *systemic involvement* or evidence of *spread of the infection*. Signs and symptoms suggesting systemic involvement or a progressive infection include: fever, malaise, cellulitis, unexplained trismus, and swelling beyond simple mucosal enlargement that affects the soft palate, floor of the mouth, or other anatomic space. Antimicrobial therapy is indicated in addition to debridement of the root canal system and drainage to contain the infection and prevent serious consequences from its spread. Patients with the above signs and symptoms should be carefully monitored on a daily basis until the infection is controlled. If there is any question about the patient's health or if the patient's condition deteriorates, consultation is advised and referral to a specialist should be considered.

Empiric selection of an antibiotic (see Table 12.3)

Penicillin Because infections of endodontic origin are polymicrobial, no single antibiotic is effective against all the strains of microorganisms. Penicillin remains the drug of choice because many of the bacteria encountered are susceptible to it and because it is well tolerated. However, the importance of a complete medical history must be emphasized because penicillin is the most common cause of drug allergies. Penicillin is effective against numerous facultative and anaerobic microorganisms. The anaerobic spectrum of penicillin includes: *Fusobacterium, Peptostreptococcus, Actinomyces,* and some *Bacteroides* sp.[18] A loading dose of 1,000 mg of penicillin VK should be orally administered, followed by 500 mg every 6 hours for 7 to 10 days. With concurrent debridement of the root canal system and drainage of purulence, significant improvement of the infection should be seen within 72 hours.

Doxycycline or minocycline These tetracyclines are broad spectrum antibiotics effective against a broad range of microorganisms. Doxycycline and minocycline are long-acting antibiotics that are active against anaerobes. A loading dose of 200 mg should be administered, followed by 100 mg every 12 hours for 7 days. Gastrointestinal upset is common. The intake of foods containing calcium or iron, or of antacids containing aluminum, does not decrease the oral absorption of doxycycline and minocycline.

Erythromycin Erythromycin has traditionally remained the antibiotic of choice for patients allergic to penicillin. It has a spectrum of activity similar to penicillin for gram-

---

Table 12.3 Primary systemic antibiotics for adjunctive treatment of endodontic infections

---

Penicillin VK
  Drug of first choice
  Confirm no allergies to penicillin

  Dosage:
  Load with 1,000 mg
  Then 500 mg every 6 h for 7–10 d

Doxycycline or minocycline
  Drug of second choice
  Gastrointestinal upset is common

  Dosage:
  Load with 200 mg
  Then 100 mg every 6 h for 7 d

Erythromycin
  Drug of choice with patients allergic to penicillin
  Gastrointestinal upset
  Not effective against some oral anaerobes
  Use enteric coated form

  Dosage:
  Load with 1,000 mg
  Then 500 mg every 6 h for 7 d

---

positive microorganisms but is *not* effective against the anaerobes usually involved in dental infections. A loading dose of 1,000 mg of enteric-coated erythromycin should be administered, followed by 500 mg every 6 hours for 7 days. A significant side effect of erythromycin is gastrointestinal upset, which subsides when the drug is discontinued.

Clindamycin Clindamycin is primarily effective against gram-positive microorganisms but is also effective against some gram-negative anaerobes, including the oral *Bacteroides* sp. Clindamycin is well distributed throughout most body tissues and reaches a concentration in bone approximating that of plasma. The usual oral adult dosage is 150 to 300 mg every 6 hours for 7 days. Food may be taken with the antibiotic to avoid stomach upset. Because clindamycin therapy has been associated with severe colitis it should be reserved for severe infections where less toxic antimicrobial agents are not appropriate. Before prescribing clindamycin, consultation with a specialist or the patient's physician is recommended.

Metronidazole Metronidazole is a synthetic antimicrobial agent that is bacteriocidal and has exceptional activity against anaerobes, including *Bacteroides, Fusobacterium, Eubacterium, Peptostreptococcus,* and *Veillonella.*[18] Although metronidazole is not the drug of choice for dental infections, it has been used extensively as an adjunct in the treatment of periodontitis and has been extremely valuable for the treatment of anaerobic infections in general when other antibiotics are ineffective or contraindicated. The usual oral dosage for anaerobic infections is 250 to 500 mg three times daily for 7 days. The most common side effect is gastrointestinal upset, which is especially provoked by alcoholic beverages. The most serious side effects are convulsive seizures and peripheral neuropathy. Before prescribing metronidazole when patients fail to respond to initial therapy, consultation with a specialist or the patient's physician is recommended.

Cephalosporins   The cephalosporins are chemically related to the penicillins with a similar spectrum of activity and produce allergies in 5% to 15% of the patients allergic to penicillin. Although cephalosporins may be used in patients who are allergic to penicillin if the patients are carefully monitored in the office after taking the first dose, **it is recommended that cephalosporins not be used in patients allergic to penicillin.** Cephalosporins have poor bone penetration and are not the drug of choice for severe anaerobic infections. Their use is limited to infections when other antibiotics are ineffective or cannot be used.

When and how to culture

Indications for microbial sampling

Medically compromised   A medically compromised patient who is not immunocompetent or a patient with a high risk of infective endocarditis should have a culture taken at the first appointment. Diabetics do not generally respond well to infections and are considered immunocompromised. Microbial sampling may be indicated for diabetics and others who are medically compromised. Identification of anaerobes or results of susceptibility tests may take several days to a couple of weeks, depending on the microorganisms involved in an infection. In addition, either the American Heart Association recommendations for prophylactic antimicrobial therapy (see chapter 17) or an antibiotic regimen specifically recommended by the patient's physician should be followed.

Persistent symptoms   A microbial sample should be taken when an otherwise healthy patient has persistent symptoms following surgical or nonsurgical root canal therapy. Persistent symptoms may include: tenderness to touch (percussion) and palpation, swelling, drainage from the root canal, or a sinus tract. Such symptoms may be associated with a pathogenic microorganism (e.g., *Actinomyces*) or gross microbial contamination.

Processing a microbial sampling

Communication with laboratory Good communication with a laboratory will ensure that the sample is properly collected, transported, cultured, and identified. Request a Gram's stain of the sample to determine what types of microorganisms are predominant. The laboratory personnel should be made aware that the culture results should reflect all of the prominent isolated microorganisms and that prominent oral species should not be considered "normal oral flora."

Sampling exudate from a root canal The tooth to be sampled must be effectively isolated with a rubber dam and the field disinfected with sodium hypochlorite or another disinfectant. Antimicrobial solutions should not be used after access to the root canal system has been made. Sterile burs and instruments are used to gain access to the pulp cavity. If exudate is present in the tooth, it may be sampled with a sterile paper point and immediately placed in a prereduced transport medium provided by a laboratory. If there is copious drainage, it may be aspirated into a sterile syringe with an 18- or 20-gauge needle. Air should be vented from the syringe and the aspirate injected into the prereduced transport medium. Some laboratories will accept the sample in the syringe if it can be transported to the laboratory within just a few minutes.

Sampling microbes from a dry root canal Use a sterile syringe to place some prereduced transport medium in the canal. A sterile endodontic instrument can be used to scrape the walls of the canal to get microorganisms into the medium. The medium in the canal can either be sampled with a sterile paper point or aspirated into a sterile syringe and then deposited in the transport medium tube.

Sampling exudate from a submucosal swelling Before an incision is made, an 18- or 20-gauge needle and syringe should be used to aspirate the exudate. After air is vented from the syringe, the needle is inserted through the sealed cap of the sample tube and the exudate is injected into prereduced transport medium. If a sample cannot be aspirated, a sample can be collected on a swab after the incision for drainage is made. Care must be taken not to contaminate the swab with saliva. The swab used should be from an anaerobic swab tube. After collecting the sample, the swab should be quickly placed into another prereduced tube for transport to the laboratory.

Identification and antibiotic susceptibility Once growth of the microorganisms is observed, colonies are subcultured both aerobically and anaerobically to determine if the isolate is facultative. The microorganisms can then be identified and antibiotic susceptibility testing undertaken to establish the minimum inhibitory concentration of the antibiotics available. Antibiotics can usually be chosen to treat anaerobic infections based on the identification of the isolates and without susceptibility testing. Because most infections of endodontic origin are polymicrobial, it is difficult to perform anaerobic susceptibility tests for all the isolated species within a short time period. Many laboratories also do not have the capability to do susceptibility testing for strict anaerobes. It is therefore recommended that antibiotics be chosen based on the microbial pattern and that susceptibility testing be performed only if the laboratory routinely tests for antibiotic susceptibility of anaerobes. A history of antibiotic usage in the previous 6 months or a failure to respond to penicillin suggests the need for a β-lactamase inhibitor (see chapters 3 and 5).

References

1. Miller, W.D. 1890. *Microorganisms of the Human Mouth*. Philadelphia: The S.S. White Dental Mfg. Co.

2. Kakehashi, S., Stanley, H.R., and Fitzgerald, R.J. 1965. The effects of surgical exposures of dental pulps in germ-free and conventional laboratory rats. *Oral Surg.* 20:340–348.

3. Allard, U., et al. 1979. Experimental infections with *Staphylococcus aureus, Streptococcus sanguis, Pseudomonas aeruginosa*, and *Bacteroides fragilis* in the jaws of dogs. *Oral Surg.* 48:454–462.

4. Sundqvist, G.K. 1976. *Bacteriologic studies of necrotic dental pulps*. Odontological Dissertation No. 7, University of Umea, Umea, Sweden.

5. Goodman, A.D. 1977. Isolation of anaerobic bacteria from the root canal systems of necrotic teeth by the use of a transport solution. *Oral Surg.* 43:766–770.

6. Baumgartner, J.C. Unpublished data.

7. Chow, A.W., Roser, S.M., and Brady, F.A. 1978. Orofacial odontogenic infections. *Ann. Intern. Med.* 88:392–402.

8. Brook, I., Grimm, S., and Kielich, R.B. 1981. Bacteriology of acute periapical abscess in children. *J. Endodontol.* 7:378–380.

9. Williams, B.L., McCann, G.F., and Schoenknecht, F.D. 1983. Bacteriology of dental abscesses of endodontic origin. *J. Clin. Microbiol.* 18:770–774.

10. Griffee, M.B., et al. 1980. The relationship of *Bacteroides melaninogenicus* to symptoms associated with pulpal necrosis. *Oral Surg.* 50:457–461.

11. Haapasalo, M., Ranta, H., and Shah, H. 1986. Black-pigmented *Bacteroides* spp. in human apical periodontitis. *Infect. Immun.* 53:149–153.

12. Sundqvist, G., Johansson, E., and Sjögren, U. 1989. Prevalence of black-pigmented *Bacteroides* species in root canal infections. *J. Endodontol.* 15:13–19.

13. Van Winkelhoff, A., Carlee, A., and de Graaff, J. 1985. *Bacteroides endodontalis* and other black-pigmented *Bacteroides* species in odontogenic abscesses. *Infect. Immun.* 49:494–497.

14. Bender, I., Seltzer, S., and Yermish, M. 1960. Incidence of bacteremias in endodontic manipulation. *Oral Surg.* 13:353–360.

15. Baumgartner, J.C., Heggers, J., and Harrison, J. 1976. The incidence of bacteremias related to endodontic procedures. I. Nonsurgical endodontics. *J. Endodontol.* 2:135–140.

16. Shulman, S.T., et al. 1984. Prevention of bacterial endocarditis. *Circulation.* 70:1123A–1127A.

17. Baumgartner, J.C., and Plack, W.F. 1982. Dental treatment and management of a patient with a prosthetic heart valve. *J. Am. Dent. Assoc.* 104:181–184.

18. Sutter, V.L., Jones, M.J., and Ghoneim, A.T. 1983. Antimicrobial susceptibilities of bacteria associated with periodontal disease. *Antimicrob. Agents Chemother.* 23:483–485.

CHAPTER 13

Antibiotics for Oral and Maxillofacial Infections

Larry J. Peterson, D.D.S., M.S.

Infections of the oral and maxillofacial region are commonly encountered by the dentist and may present a management problem. Most of these infections are minor and can be easily managed by administering appropriate antibiotics and performing minor surgical procedures. Such infections arise as the result of severe periodontal disease or of dental decay that has caused a necrotic dental pulp. On rare occasions these infections become severe and will require management by a specialist, sometimes in the hospital setting. Following are guidelines to manage minor orofacial and odontogenic infection in the office setting using a combination of antibiotics and surgery.

Microbiology of odontogenic infection

Carefully performed microbiological studies that have been done over the last decade have clearly established the etiological bacteria for odontogenic infections.[1-3] Most of these studies have been performed on pus aspirated percutaneously from an odontogenic abscess. Both facultative aerobes and anaerobic bacteria are grown. Strict aerobes are rarely found in the oral cavity and most of the oral bacteria that are grown in air are facultative, meaning that they are able to grow with and without oxygen. The facultative bacteria are primarily streptococci, but a wide variety of other organisms are also found. The anaerobic bacteria are primarily anaerobic gram-positive cocci such as *Peptococcus* and *Peptostreptococcus* sp. and anaerobic gram-negative bacilli such as *Fusobacterium* and *Bacteroides* sp.

The facultative–anaerobic distribution of the bacteria is somewhat variable. In approximately 5% of the situations, only facultative bacteria are found. Pure anaerobic cultures are obtained in about 35% of the patients, while the remaining 60% have both facultative and anaerobic bacteria.

Because anaerobic bacteria tend to produce pus with greater frequency than facultative bacteria, the abscess stage of the infection, which tends to be later, is caused primarily by anaerobic bacteria. The earlier stage of an infection (that is, the portion

---

Table 13.1   Natural course of odontogenic infections

Initial stage: Cellulitis

Phase 1
Erythema
Diffuse swelling
Pain
Doughy consistency

Phase 2
Swelling increased
Hard consistency
Indurated
Significant pain
Usually elevated temperature

Second stage: Abscess

Well-defined borders
Pus accumulation in tissues
Fluctuant to palpation

Third stage: Sinus tract

Abscess ruptures to produce a draining sinus tract

---

with no pus) is most likely caused by facultative bacteria such as streptococci. This concept has been fairly well established by experimental infections in animals, as well as in the clinical management of odontogenic infections.

Natural course of odontogenic infections (see **Table 13.1**)

When bacteria gain access to the underlying tissue and an infection becomes established, it follows a relatively predictable course depending on the type of bacteria, its inherent invasiveness, and the patient's host resistance. Certain bacteria, like streptococci, tend to spread rapidly but not to form pus. Other bacteria, such as the anaerobic bacteria, tend to have a slow, insidious onset and produce pus.

Initial stage—cellulitis   The initial phase that occurs when bacteria gain access to the underlying tissues as the result of odontogenic sources is usually a cellulitis stage. A cellulitis is usually acute, has diffuse borders, and does not produce pus. In its early stages it has a soft, doughy consistency to palpation. The overlying skin is likely to appear erythematous, and the patient usually has significant pain. As the cellulitis progresses, the swelling becomes larger and harder until it becomes indurated. Induration is the result of extravasation of fluid from the vascular space into the interstitial tissue, producing tension in the tissue that compresses blood vessels and thereby compromises the vascular supply to the local area. When the cellulitis is in the indurated stage, the patient almost always has significant pain and a high temperature. At this point the infection is usually quite serious.

The bacteria that cause the cellulitis stage are usually facultative bacteria such as streptococci. Therefore, antibiotic management of a cellulitis should be primarily directed at facultative bacteria.

Second stage—abscess The second stage of the infection is the abscess stage. At this point the body is able to mobilize its defenses sufficiently to wall off the infection and limit its spread. The result of the accumulation of the polymorphonuclear leukocytes is the production of pus. By definition an abscess is a localized collection of pus within a tissue space. The abscess is more chronic in nature than the cellulitis and frequently has well-defined borders. **The abscess will feel fluctuant to palpation, the result of accumulation of pus within the tissue.** While some abscesses are serious, usually the presence of a well-defined chronic abscess indicates that the host defenses have been sufficiently potent to wall off and contain the infectious process.

The bacteria responsible for abscess formation are predominately anaerobic bacteria. Although facultative bacteria such as streptococci are frequently found in pus specimens from abscesses, their role in the abscess process is relatively minor.

In serious odontogenic infections that appear to be primarily an advanced stage cellulitis with induration, it is very common to find small or even sizeable areas of abscess formation. That is to say, an abscess frequently will exist within a large area of cellulitis. In these situations, both anaerobic and facultative bacteria are playing important roles.

Third stage—sinus tract The third stage of the infectious process is the formation of a sinus tract. In these situations the abscess ruptures intraorally, or occasionally extraorally, and a chronic draining sinus tract is established. As long as this sinus tract continues to drain there will be no overt signs of infection, such as swelling, pain, or temperature. If the patient is treated with antibiotics, the sinus tract will usually cease to drain, but after withdrawal of the antibiotic the sinus tract will open again. The method of treatment in this situation is to remove the source of the infection, either by endodontic therapy or by tooth extraction.

In summary, odontogenic infections begin with invasion of a mixed bacterial flora into the underlying tissue. In the early stages the facultative bacteria such as streptococci are predominant and a cellulitis is established. If the infection is treated at this point, there will not be a progression to an abscess. If the infection is left untreated, the cellulitis will progress from the soft doughy swelling to a harder, indurated swelling. During this process the oxidation-reduction potential in the local tissue becomes such that the hypoxic, acidotic environment favors the overgrowth of anaerobic bacteria and the lack of growth of facultative bacteria.[1] This change in the bacterial population, coupled with the increased response in the host, will result in abscess formation.

The cellulitis then can be characterized as a primarily facultative infection that tends to be rapidly progressive and spreads, does not produce pus, and can become quite serious if not treated promptly. The abscess can be characterized as being primarily an

---

Table 13.2   Spread of odontogenic infections

Primary determinants of direction of spread
- Thickness of overlying bone
- Position of muscle attachments

Maxilla

Most common spread: facial

Other spread: buccal space if infection perforates bone superior to attachment of buccinator muscle

Mandibular anterior teeth and premolars

Most common spread: buccal vestibule

Mandibular posterior teeth

Most common spread: submandibular space

Spread producing major risks

Involvement of fascial spaces posteriorly and inferiorly into the neck

---

anaerobic infection, which is usually chronic, has more well-defined margins, is fluctuant, and is filled with pus. These two stages of the infection are treated quite differently, as will be discussed in subsequent sections.

Spread of infection (see **Table 13.2**)   Once an infection has been established in the periapical area, it will spread through the bone and involve the adjacent tissues. The primary determinants of the direction of the spread of the infection are the thickness of the overlying bone and the position of the muscle attachment in relationship to the infection. In the maxilla, the labial-buccal cortical bone is quite thin; consequently, almost all maxillary infections spread to the facial aspect, almost always resulting in a vestibular abscess. However, if the infection erodes through the bone superior to the attachment of the buccinator muscle, as it does occasionally in the molar region, a buccal space infection may result.

In the mandible, the labial-buccal bone is likewise relatively thin around the anterior teeth and around the premolars. Therefore, the most common location for infection in those situations is in the buccal vestibule. However, in the posterior region, the lingual cortical plate is thinner, and the attachment of the mylohyoid muscle is relatively high in relationship to the apex of the molars; therefore, the result is a submandibular space infection.

Infection from these spaces can continue posteriorly and inferiorly into the neck and possibly even into the thorax. Infections that involve fascial spaces should be treated vigorously, and the patient should be referred to a specialist early for combined antibiotic and surgical treatment.

Depressed host defenses (see chapter 18)

Patients with odontogenic infections who have a decrease in their ability to mobilize normal host defenses will have increased need for early and more aggressive antibiotic and surgical treatment. A variety of conditions will cause compromise in these host defenses and need to be identified in the patient's history so that proper modification of treatment can be made.

Chemotherapy   One of the most common causes of depressed host defenses is patients who are receiving chemotherapy for treatment of a variety of cancers. Cancer chemotherapeutic agents kill rapidly dividing cells, such as are found in cancer, but also those that are found in bone marrow. The result is that the patient has fewer polymorphonuclear leukocytes to combat infection.

Metabolic diseases   A second common cause is severe uncontrolled metabolic diseases, such as diabetes, uremia, and alcoholism. These metabolic diseases, when uncompensated and severe in nature, result in depressed leukocyte function and depressed immunoglobulin and complement function.

Organ transplants   A third cause is patients who have received organ transplants such as kidneys, livers, or hearts who are receiving cyclosporin for immunosuppression to increase chances of the graft survival. This immunosuppressive drug decreases the immune system, thereby prolonging graft life but also making the patient more likely to develop an infection.

Myeloproliferative diseases   A final cause of depressed host defenses is the group of diseases referred to as the myeloproliferative diseases, such as leukemia and lymphoma. They result in poorly functioning leukocytes that make the patient more susceptible to infection.

   In summary, the patient with depressed host defenses will have impaired antibacterial defenses, an increased risk of infection, and an increased rate of spread when infection occurs. Because there is lack of adequate support from the defenses, these infections are also more difficult to treat when they occur. The antibiotic used in these patients should be bactericidal.

Dental spectrum antibiotics (see chapter 5)

Because the microbiology of odontogenic infections has been carefully defined (that is, almost always being caused by facultative streptococci and anaerobic gram-positive cocci and anaerobic gram-negative rods), the proper choice of an antibiotic without culture and sensitivity can usually be made in these infections. The antibacterial spectrum of a variety of antibiotics will kill or slow the growth of the causative organism. Following are the antibiotics most commonly used in managing odontogenic infections.

Penicillin

Orally administered penicillin V is the drug of choice for most mild to moderate odontogenic infections. It is a bactericidal drug that kills streptococci and most oral anaerobic bacteria. It has low toxicity and is tolerated well by most patients. Although approximately 3% of the patient population is allergic to penicillin, severe allergic reactions are relatively uncommon when this drug is administered orally. It is also a drug of choice for the prophylaxis of subacute bacterial endocarditis in the nonallergic patient (see chapter 17).

Extended-spectrum penicillins

Biochemical alteration of the basic structure of the penicillin molecule has resulted in a variety of penicillin-like antibiotics. These antibiotics have extended antibacterial activity and presumably are more useful for infections. **Ampicillin** and **amoxicillin** are two commonly recommended antibiotics that have an increased spectrum. However, they have a more limited additional activity against streptococci or oral anaerobes than penicillin V. Their extended spectrum is almost exclusively in the area of gram-negative aerobic rods such as *Hemophilus influenzae*, *Escherichia coli*, *Salmonella*, *Shigella*, and *Proteus* organisms. Therefore, there is essentially no indication in the management of odontogenic infections for these extended-spectrum antibiotics. If a culture and sensitivity obtained in a difficult infection reveal that the causative organism is *H. influenzae*, then amoxicillin might be considered an effective antibiotic in its management.

Cephalosporin antibiotics

An antibiotic family with a similar molecular structure to penicillin is the group of antibiotics known as the **cephalosporins.** Like penicillin, cephalosporins are bactericidal and have a low toxicity. Generally their antibiotic spectrum is broader than penicillin and they tend to be more expensive than penicillin. There are a large number of cephalosporins available, but only a few can be taken orally. The two that are most popular in dentistry are, **cephalexin** (Keflex®) and **cefadroxil** (Duricef®). These antibiotics are effective against streptococci, staphylococci, oral anaerobes, and some gram-negative aerobic rods such as *E. coli* and *Proteus* and *Klebsiella* sp. Cephalosporins have been shown to produce allergic reactions in 5% to 15% of the patients allergic to penicillin, and in general those agents should not be used in patients with a history of allergic reaction to penicillin. In spite of these concerns, cephalosporins may be useful in the penicillin-allergic patient who has compromised host-defense mechanisms and requires a bactericidal antibiotic, if the patient is carefully monitored in the office after taking the first dose. In general this approach to the use of cephalosporins should not be considered except under the supervision of a specialist and/or physician who is comfortable with the management of acute allergic reactions.

Erythromycin

Erythromycin is a bacteriostatic antibiotic that is effective against streptococci, staphylococci, and some oral anaerobes. It is also effective against several other organisms that rarely cause odontogenic infections. It is useful primarily by the oral route and has a relatively low toxicity when taken at doses below 2 g per day. Its main limitation is that it is not useful for more serious infections, because of the dose limitation; also, there exists moderate bacterial resistance to this antibiotic. The primary indication of erythromycin is for treatment of mild odontogenic infections in healthy patients who are allergic to penicillin.

Clindamycin

Clindamycin is effective against streptococci, staphylococci, and essentially all anaerobic bacteria. It is bacteriostatic in most situations and has a higher toxicity. It is substantially more expensive than penicillin, therefore it is usually not considered as a first-line drug for odontogenic infections. However, it has been found to be a useful and effective drug in chronic low-grade infections that have been resistant to previous treatment with penicillin or erythromycin. Diarrhea may occur in 20% to 30% of the patients treated with clindamycin, but it is reversible and subsides rapidly with discontinuance of therapy.

Tetracycline

The family of tetracycline antibiotics has been available since the mid-1950s. Its original spectrum included streptococci, staphylococci, oral anaerobes, and a variety of gram-negative aerobic rods. However, because of its wide use and because it is a bacteriostatic drug, there is a high degree of bacterial resistance at this time. The drug has relatively mild toxicities, and it is inexpensive. Its main indication in the maxillofacial area would be a mild odontogenic infection in a patient who has severe allergy to penicillin and the cephalosporins and cannot tolerate erythromycin.

Metronidazole

Metronidazole is bactericidal against all anaerobic bacteria but has absolutely no activity against facultative bacteria such as streptococci. Therefore, metronidazole is an effective antibiotic for managing chronic infections that are caused primarily by anaerobic bacteria, but it has little or no indication in the cellulitis stage of an infection.

Table 13.3 Antibiotic selection summary for odontogenic infections

---

Drug of choice: Penicillin V

If patient is penicillin allergic:

- Erythromycin—bacteriostatic
- Cephalosporin—bactericidal; *note:* may produce allergic reactions in 5%–15% of the patients allergic to penicillin
- Tetracyclines—bacteriostatic; use if allergic to penicillins and cephalosporins and cannot tolerate erythromycin

Chronic infection, inadequate response to penicillin:

- Clindamycin
- Metronidazole
- Metronidazole + penicillin in more severe infections

It is well absorbed orally, has a mild toxicity level, and is inexpensive. Its primary indication is to treat chronic anaerobic infections. Occasionally it is used in combination with penicillin or a cephalosporin for managing a severe fascial space infection.

Antibiotic selection summary (see **Table 13.3**)

The selection of an antibiotic for the initial management of an odontogenic infection can be made with great predictability because the antibacterial pattern has been so well described. Penicillin remains the drug of choice for odontogenic infections. An oral cephalosporin such as **cephalexin** is useful in patients who are allergic to penicillin and who require a bactericidal drug. (*Caution*: 5% to 15% of the patients who are allergic to penicillin will have cross-reacting allergies to cephalosporins such as cephalexin.) **Erythromycin** is effective for a mild odontogenic infection in a patient who is allergic to penicillin and who does not require a bactericidal antibiotic. **Clindamycin** is primarily useful in a chronic infection thought to be caused by anaerobic bacteria that has not responded to penicillin. **Metronidazole** is an effective drug for treating a chronic, well-established abscess, and perhaps in combination with penicillin for a serious infection. **Tetracycline** has a very limited role in the management of odontogenic infections.

Principles of therapy (see **Table 13.4**)

The approach to managing odontogenic infections should be systematic and logical so that important pieces of information are not omitted and the progress of the patient is carefully monitored.[4]

Table 13.4   Principles of managing odontogenic infections

Step 1: Determine severity

- History of onset and progression
- Physical examination of area
  - *(1)* character and size of swelling
  - *(2)* presence of trismus

Step 2: Evaluate host defenses

- Diseases that compromise the host
- Medications that compromise the host

Step 3: Surgical treatment

- Remove the cause of infection
- Drain pus
- Relieve pressure

Step 4: Antibiotic choice

- Determine:
  - *(1)* most likely causative organisms based on history
  - *(2)* host defense status
  - *(3)* allergy history
  - *(4)* previous drug history
- Prescribe drug properly

Step 5: Followup

- Confirm treatment response
- Evaluate for side effects and secondary infections

Determine severity   The first step is to determine the severity of the infection. This will be done by taking a thorough history of the onset and progress of the infection as well as by physical examination. The history of pain and the spread of the pain from the local area are important to note. It is also important to note the rate of progression of the infection. An infection that progresses rapidly over hours will be much more serious than an infection that develops and spreads over a period of days or weeks. On physical examination one should note the swelling, both from a quantitative point of view as well as a qualitative. That is, how large is the swelling, and how does it feel to palpation? A soft, doughy, early cellulitis probably can be managed by antibiotic therapy alone and by treating the offending tooth. An indurated cellulitis or a fluctuant abscess will require incision and drainage as well as antibiotic therapy. The presence of trismus (limitation of opening) is also important. Trismus usually indicates that there is involvement of the muscles of mastication and therefore is a serious sign.

Evaluate host defenses   The next step is to evaluate the patient's host defenses. Diseases and medications that were mentioned earlier need to be identified. If the patient has any of the factors that may decrease host defenses, the doctor needs to be aware that the infection may spread more rapidly and has an increased chance of becoming severe. Bactericidal antibiotics will be necessary, removal of the offending tooth is more likely to be indicated than conservative endodontic therapy, and early referral to a specialist and early hospitalization will be more frequently indicated in patients with compromised host defenses.

Surgical treatment   The first treatment modality in managing infections is to treat the patient surgically. The three primary goals of surgical treatment are to remove the cause (i.e., the necrotic pulp of the tooth), drain pus that has accumulated in any abscess space, and relieve pressure in the indurated cellulitis situation. Surgical treatment may simply be to open a tooth and remove the necrotic pulp, or it may be complex as with extensive incision and drainage of the soft tissue involved in the infection.

Antibiotic choice   An antibiotic is chosen that will be effective against the likely causative organisms. As discussed before, empiric therapy is usually correct. When deciding which antibiotic to prescribe, such factors as host defenses, allergy status, and previous drug history are important. In general, a narrow-spectrum antibiotic is preferred over a broad-spectrum antibiotic so that the fewest number of normal host bacteria will be altered as possible. Obviously the least toxic drug should be chosen preferentially. The doctor should also be aware of the drug cost, because two drugs that are equally effective and equally toxic may vary dramatically in their cost to the patient.

Antibiotic administration   Once an antibiotic is selected it should be given properly. This means that the drug should be given by the proper route, usually the oral route in mild to moderate odontogenic infections, in the proper dose, and at the proper dosage interval. The latter two factors are well delineated in reference books, package inserts, and in the *Physicians' Desk Reference*.[5] The antibiotic should be given for an adequate length of time, usually for at least 2 days after the major clinical symptoms disappear. In most mild odontogenic infections that have appropriate antibiotic and surgical care there will be a dramatic improvement within 2 days and major resolution within 4 or 5 days. Therefore, the usual prescription would be written for 7 days.

Followup   The patient should be followed carefully after the initial appointment. The doctor would usually see the patient the following day or at least talk with him or her by telephone. The major goal at this time is to look for a treatment response. If the patient is treated with antibiotics alone, there might be little improvement but the patient should not be worse. By the second or third day the patient's condition should begin to significantly improve. However, if the patient received both surgical treatment and antibiotic treatment, by the first postoperative day he or she will feel much better.

Side effects and secondary infection   The doctor will also need to examine and follow the patient for allergic reactions, toxicity reactions, and side effects typical for the antibiotics being given. For example, erythromycin frequently causes gastrointestinal distress as an expected side effect. Patients can be advised to take their antibiotic with small amounts of food, which will tend to make the drug more tolerable. The doctor will also need to watch for secondary infections. The most common secondary infection that occurs as the result of management of odontogenic infection would be oral or vaginal candidiasis. This most commonly would occur after 10 to 14 days of antibiotic therapy (see chapter 8 on antifungal therapy).

Wound infection prophylaxis

Some patients, especially those with compromised host defenses, will need to have antibiotics to prevent infection in the operative wound when surgical procedures are performed in the mouth. The guidelines for antibiotic prophylaxis in this situation have been well defined.[6,7]

Choose correct antibiotic   The first guideline is to choose the correct antibiotic. For surgery in the mouth, the antibiotic chosen should be the same one used for therapy, that is, penicillin or an alternative drug, depending on the patient's allergic status. It is best also to use a bactericidal drug for prophylaxis.

Plasma level   The second guideline is that the plasma level of the antibiotic should be high, higher than for treatment of infection. This means that the dose of the antibiotic should be twice the usual dose of an antibiotic. If, for example, the normal dose of penicillin is 500 mg, the prophylactic dose would be 1 g.

Correct administration   The third guideline is to time the antibiotic administration correctly. **The first dose should be given before the surgery begins.** If the surgery is long (i.e., over 2 hours) an additional dose should be given in the middle of the operation.

Antibiotic exposure   The final guideline for effective use of prophylaxis is to use the shortest antibiotic exposure that is effective. Many animal and human clinical studies have defined this very well; the universal conclusion of these reports is that the final dose of the antibiotic should be given at the end of the surgical procedure. Therefore, for most surgery done in the office setting, a patient should be given 1 g of penicillin 1 hour before the operation is begun and a second dose of 1 g of penicillin before the patient leaves the office. If the procedure lasts for 3 hours, an interim dose of 1 g could be given approximately 2 hours after the first dose.

Special considerations

In the course of dental practice, clinical situations present where the need for antibiotics is not clear. These situations are both therapeutic and prophylactic.

Sinus perforations   When extracting teeth from a maxillary arch with a large maxillary sinus, the possibility exists that a small piece of bone may be removed with the root, resulting in a perforation of the maxillary sinus. The most common tooth involved in such inadvertent perforations is the maxillary first molar. When such events occur, attention is directed at preventing the formation of a chronic fistulous tract, or communication, between the maxillary sinus and the oral cavity. Almost all perforations are small and in fact a large number go unrecognized. If the perforation is large, as when the bone encasing all three roots of the maxillary first molar is removed with the tooth, a more aggressive surgical approach to close this perforation must be done. In this situation a referral to an oral and maxillofacial surgeon would be indicated.

For the small perforation, a relatively well-established regimen will prevent the formation of a chronic fistula. Every effort is made to maintain a proper blood clot, sometimes with the use of Gelfoam, Surgicel, or sutures over the top of the socket. Sinus precautions are recommended to the patient, which include avoiding sneezing, sucking through a straw, and doing other maneuvers that would create a differential pressure between the mouth and sinus. Sinus decongestants are frequently prescribed as well. Most clinicians also prefer to prescribe an antibiotic to decrease the chance for an infection, although it is very unlikely. The bacteria that would cause such an infection would primarily be the normal mouth bacteria; therefore, penicillin would be the drug of choice, with erythromycin being the drug of second choice in the penicillin-allergic patient. If the decision is made to use antibiotics, they should be started as soon as possible after the perforation is noted and continued for approximately 5 days.

Avulsed teeth   Management of avulsed teeth is a complex problem that requires a variety of different decisions be made. Fundamental to success is the replacement of the avulsed tooth back into the socket as quickly as possible and stabilization of the avulsed teeth to adjacent teeth in such a way as to allow some mild amount of movement. Care should be taken to avoid injury to the root and cementum of the tooth, so as to prevent areas of resorption and/or ankylosis. The issue as to whether antibiotics should be used or not is again one of clinical opinion. While no controlled studies have been performed to define whether antibiotics should be prescribed for such patients, it is common clinical practice that antibiotics should be used. The drug of choice in these settings is penicillin, with erythromycin in the penicillin-allergic patient. The antibiotics should be started as soon as possible and continued for 5 to 7 days. In some situations when there has been more soft tissue and bone injury, the clinician may decide to use antibiotics for a longer period of time.

Osteomyelitis   Osteomyelitis of the jaws is an infrequent occurrence, but when it does occur it usually has several common predisposing parameters. Osteomyelitis is seen primarily in patients who are debilitated by systemic disease, the most common one being alcoholism. Second, there is usually some traumatic event that is the immediate precipitating cause. The most common is fracture of the mandible, followed by extraction of the tooth, which leads to a nonhealing dry socket. The diagnosis and management of osteomyelitis of the jaw is a complex topic and would require an extensive discussion to provide even basic information. Generally, however, osteomyelitis causes pain, draining sinus tracts, either intraorally or extraorally, destruction of bone that is obvious on the radiograph, and frequently is very difficult to eradicate. Aggressive surgical intervention and precise antibiotic choices are necessary for prompt resolution of this disease. The antibiotic of choice in these situations is primarily a drug that is effective against the anaerobic bacteria of the mouth and that also has effectiveness against *Streptococcus*. While *Staphylococcus* has been implicated as a causative bacteria in osteomyelitis of the jaws, recent investigations have established that it is not a major causative organism. Therefore, a drug like clindamycin, which is excellent against anaerobes, would be one of the first line drugs. Penicillin, alone or in combination with metronidazole, may also be useful for the management of osteomyelitis of the jaws. Most commonly this infection would be managed by a specialist such as an oral and maxillofacial surgeon.

Dry socket   The postoperative complication known as "dry socket" or "alveolar osteitis" occurs in approximately 10% of patients who have mandibular third molars removed. This complication is most likely the result of a bacterial-induced lysis of the blood clot, which results in exposed bone and moderate to severe pain. Dry socket can best be prevented through copious intraoperative irrigation. Topical antibiotics (i.e., placement of a small amount of antibiotic directly in the socket at the end of a procedure) may reduce the incidence by approximately 50%. There is also evidence that preoperative and postoperative rinsing with **chlorhexidine** may reduce the incidence of dry socket. Once this complication has occurred, the role for antibiotics is essentially nonexistent. Irrigation of the socket to remove loose debris and placement of a sedative dressing are all that is required for its management.

Pericoronitis   The partially erupted third molar will frequently have a soft tissue operculum, which may give rise to that special periodontal infection known as *pericoronitis*. In this situation, the deep periodontal pocket caused by the operculum becomes infected and results in mild to severe infections. If the patient presents for treatment when the symptoms are very localized (i.e., local pain and swelling without trismus or extraoral swelling or temperature), the most effective method of management is to irrigate the periodontal pocket with **hydrogen peroxide, saline,** or **chlorhexidine.** Occasionally, removal of the hypererupted maxillary third molar is of great benefit as well. Antibiotics are not necessary in these mild situations. If the patient does not present for treatment until there is trismus, extraoral swelling, and temperature, irrigation and removal of the maxillary third molar will need to be supplemented by administration of antibiotics. The drug of choice in this situation continues to be **penicillin,** with alternative drugs being **erythromycin** and **cephalexin.**

Routine extractions   There is frequently concern about whether patients should receive antibiotics for routine extraction of teeth. This is almost never necessary in the patient with normal, intact host-defense mechanisms. Only when the patient has a history of diseases or drug usage such as cancer chemotherapeutic agents, which would depress host defenses, should antibiotics be used prophylactically for routine extractions.

Impacted third molars   A similar concern exists about the removal of impacted third molars. As with other dentoalveolar surgery, if the patient is healthy, prophylactic antibiotics are *not* necessary for routine third molar extraction. If the patient has an acute pericoronitis, administration of short-term prophylactic antibiotics may be of some benefit in preventing postoperative infection. However, if the pericoronitis is very mild, or if it has been resolved with irrigation and/or antibiotic therapy in the time period preceding the extraction, then antibiotics are not necessary.

References

1. Aderhold, L., Konthe, H., and Frenkel, G. 1981. The bacteriology of dentogenous pyogenic infections. *Oral Surg.* 52:583.
2. Bartlett, J.G., and O'Keefe, P. 1979. The bacteriology of perimandibular space infections. *J. Oral Surg.* 37:407.
3. Labriola, J.D., Mascaro, J., and Alpert, B. 1983. The microbiologic flora of orofacial abscesses. *J. Oral Maxillofac. Surg.* 41:711.
4. Peterson, L.J. 1988. Principles of management and prevention of odontogenic infections. Chapter 16. *In* L.J. Peterson (ed.) *Contemporary Oral and Maxillofacial Surgery.* St. Louis: The C. V. Mosby Co.
5. *Physicians' Desk Reference.* 1986. Oradell, N.J.: Medical Economics Co., Inc.
6. Conover, M.S., Kaban, L.B., and Mulliken, J.B. 1985. Antibiotic prophylaxis for major maxillocraniofacial surgery. *J. Oral Maxillofac. Surg.* 43:865.
7. Peterson, L.J. (In press.) Antibiotic prophylaxis against wound infections in oral and maxillofacial surgery. *J. Oral. Maxillofac. Surg.*

CHAPTER 14

Pediatric Considerations

Robert Lindemann, D.D.S.

Qualities of the young patient

Pediatric antibiotic therapy shares many of the general principles that have been applied to adults in the preceding chapters. The child, though, cannot always be considered a small adult for treatment purposes. Understanding differences in metabolism, anatomy, and cognitive processes will enable the dentist to treat the child confidently and successfully.

Cognition During the early stages of their development, children are busy collecting the experiential knowledge that will be incorporated in the creation of their unique personalities. They frequently need understanding and extra patience from the dentist to make dental visits as pleasant as possible. This is especially true if the child presents with an infection or condition that elicits pain or is uncomfortable.

Metabolism The child is fortunate to have the resiliency of youth, yet it is important to remain aware of the potential dangers of unchecked orofacial infection to the child patient. Infection can spread quickly with dramatic changes in signs and symptoms.

Microflora At their first dental encounters, pediatric patients with primary dentition present with many of the same indigenous bacteria found in the normal microflora of adults. Children undergo progressive addition of oral bacteria after their first exposures during passage through the maternal birth canal and with the eruption of primary teeth.[1,2]

Occasions when antibiotic therapy will benefit the child will be discussed in this chapter. The variety of systemic conditions together with new advances in medical treatment of those conditions necessitates consultation with the pediatrician. The goals of this chapter are twofold: *(1)* to reinforce the application of appropriate antibiotic therapy for the child, and *(2)* to alert the reader to the required modifications of therapy.

Table 14.1 Average doses recommended for children

Actual doses are based on infection severity, child's age, and renal and hepatic clearances

Antibiotic	Usual oral dose
Ampicillin	50–100 mg/kg/d in 4 divided doses up to 250 mg/dose
Cephalexin	25–50 mg/kg/d in 4–6 divided doses
Clindamycin	8–25 mg/kg/d in 3–4 divided doses
Erythromycin	30–40 mg/kg/d in 4 divided doses (maximum of 2 g/d)
Penicillin V	25–50 mg/kg/d in 4 divided doses

Pediatric antibiotic therapy: Indications and treatment

Acute odontogenic infections

Dangers Wide marrow spaces in children can allow permanent tooth germs and critical growth centers of the jaws to be threatened by intraosseous infection.[3] Children are also susceptible to the life-threatening consequences of rapidly spreading odontogenic infections, which include: cavernous sinus thrombosis, brain abscess, septicemia, airway obstruction, and mediastinitis.[4] Use of antibiotics is therefore advised, concomitant with the primary treatment of pulpectomy or extraction to eliminate the source of the infection.

Penicillin The same culture techniques as for adults (see chapters 3 and 4) should be performed in conjunction with the administration of the antibiotic most likely to succeed. **Penicillin V** is the drug of choice because of the effectiveness of oral administration; see **Table 14.1** for recommended dosages. To achieve a high serum and tissue level, penicillin V should be prescribed for a minimum of 7 to 10 days. Compliance should be stressed to the responsible adult and to the young patient.

Penicillin allergy Children with documented penicillin allergy can be prescribed **erythromycin** or **clindamycin** for the treatment of *acute* odontogenic infections. Recommended erythromycin and clindamycin dosages are listed in **Table 14.1**. Discussion with the patient's physician is recommended when prescribing clindamycin.

Periapical abscess Recent clinical research has implicated anaerobic microorganisms in the etiology of acute periapical abscess in children.[5] This discovery was made possible by meticulous sample techniques that avoided contamination with normal

173

flora. Because these anaerobes have been associated with serious infections arising from an oral focus, appropriate antimicrobial therapy is indicated. Fortunately, most of the anaerobic pathogens isolated from the abscesses are sensitive to penicillin. However, patients who do not show signs of improvement after instituting penicillin therapy may have beta-lactamase-producing organisms, possibly *Bacteroides* sp.[6] Antimicrobial agents effective against these strains such as Augmentin® or cefoxitin may be required in serious cases.[5] In conjunction with judicious antimicrobial therapy, dental surgical intervention may also be indicated.

Severe infections   Severe infections require more aggressive treatment, including parenteral administration of antibiotics and, in extreme cases, hospitalization. Close cooperation between the dentist and pediatrician is essential. The value of initial cultures from the odontogenic abscess becomes critical in those cases that do not respond to therapy, where the failure may be caused by the development of resistant strains.

Chemoprophylaxis

Bacteremia   It has been firmly established that bacteremias do occur in children following dental prophylaxis and extraction of normal and diseased primary or permanent teeth.[7-9] Children require antibiotic prophylaxes for the same reasons adults do. These include most congenital heart diseases, rheumatic or acquired valvular heart disease, and prosthetic heart valves or vessels[10,11] (see chapter 17).
   Antibiotics are not necessary during the spontaneous exfoliation of primary teeth or the simple adjustment of orthodontic appliances.

AHA guidelines   The 1985 Chapter 13 American Heart Association report (see chapter 17) lists recommendations for the prevention of bacterial endocarditis. Adjustments according to the child's weight may need to be made.[10]
   It is important to remember that AHA guidelines are recommendations only. Close cooperation between dentist and pediatrician is essential for optimal prophylaxis. Keeping current on changing AHA regimens is the best way to prevent the high morbidity and mortality of bacterial endocarditis.[12]

Resistance   A careful history of antibiotic therapy should be elicited in those patients requiring chemoprophylaxis. Recent history of penicillin or erythromycin therapy will alert the practitioner to the possibility of resistant organisms. With children receiving frequent regimens of antibiotics for childhood illnesses, close monitoring becomes even more critical to prevent untoward sequelae of infection by those resistant strains.[13]

Periodontal disease

Local debridement remains the major treatment for most periodontal diseases in children. However, in the clinical management of localized juvenile periodontitis, tetracycline therapy may enhance success. A combined therapy of surgery and systemic antibiotics is recommended[14] (see chapter 11).

Trauma

Pediatric patients with face lacerations, through-and-through lip lacerations, puncture wounds, dog bites, or electrical burns of the orofacial complex should receive antibiotics in addition to meticulous surgical management. Consultation and/or referral to an oral surgeon or emergency room is indicated in most cases. Tetanus immunization history must be considered.[4]

Special considerations

Problems swallowing pills   Children, like some adults, often have difficulty swallowing capsules or tablets. Elixirs of penicillin V are available in dosages of 125 mg/5 mL and 250 mg/5 mL, in either 100- or 200-mL bottles. Erythromycin is available in two oral suspensions as well: 200 mg/5 mL and 400 mg/5 mL, both in pint bottles. They are flavored for palatability. Clindamycin is available in flavored granules for oral solution in the equivalent of 75 mg in each 5 mL (100- or 200-mL reconstituted bottles).

Noncompliance   It may be necessary to question compliance in some children who do not respond favorably to antibiotic treatment. A child who refuses to accept his or her medications, vomits shortly after ingestion, or is suspected of removing the tablet after it is administered is a candidate for the parenteral route. Fortunately, noncompliance is unusual, especially with flavored elixir forms.

Childhood systemic diseases   Many childhood diseases have orofacial manifestations (chicken pox, measles, mumps) and should be considered in a differential diagnosis before prescribing an antibiotic regimen for a problem of presumed odontogenic or periodontal etiology.

Chronic systemic disease   Certain special circumstances of systemic disease in pediatric patients require consideration. The **immunosuppressed** child is susceptible to infection and should be given antibiotic prophylaxis before dental manipulation.[15,16] As an adjunct, 0.12% chlorhexidine gluconate rinse (Peridex®) may be effective in reducing dental plaque bacteria. Clotrimazole (Mycelex) troches can be used to eliminate *Candida* infections frequently reported in the immunocompromised host (see chapter 18). Similarly, the chronic **renal failure** patient (possibly on dialysis or post-transplant) is also at risk to infection from dental sources.[17,18] Attention should be given to reducing the potential for an oral focus of infection in these cases. Consultation with the patient's physician is necessary to maximize antibiotic prophylaxis.

Judicious home care and regular dental examinations help reduce the threat of infection in the **diabetic** child. Some pediatricians believe that antibiotics are warranted before surgical procedures.

Children with **Down's syndrome** have an associated 40% incidence of congenital heart defects. Those patients with positive findings after a physical exam are candidates for chemoprophylaxis.[19] Croll et al.[20] have reported the need for antibiotic prophylaxis for the **hydrocephalic** dental patient with a ventriculo-peritoneal or ventriculovenous shunt. They have proposed a subjectively derived protocol modeled after the regimen used at the time of shunt surgery.

Tretracycline staining Children are susceptible to tetracycline staining of their primary and permanent dentition when the drug is prescribed during critical developmental periods. The first of these periods is approximately 4 months in utero to 9 months postpartum for primary incisors and canines. The second sensitive period is from 3 to 5 months postpartum until about the seventh year for permanent incisors and canines.[21] An alternative antibiotic should be given to preclude unsightly staining. If this is not possible, research has shown that the tretracycline analogs **chlortetracycline** and **oxytetracycline** stain the teeth less.[22] Recent reports demonstrate that minocycline, a tetracycline derivative used in the treatment of acne, has been associated with adult-onset tooth discoloration.[23,24]

References

1. Minah, G.E. 1981. Dental plaque. *In* D.J. Forrester (ed.) *Pediatric Dental Medicine*. Philadelphia: Lea & Febiger.

2. Smith, D.S. 1982. Antibiotic usage. *In* R.E. Stewart et al. (eds.) *Pediatric Dentistry: Scientific Foundations and Clinical Practice*. St. Louis: The C.V. Mosby Co.

3. McCallum, C. 1973. Oral surgery for children. *In* S.B. Finn (ed.) *Clinical Pedodontics*. 4th ed. Philadelphia: W.B. Saunders Co.

4. Sanders, B. 1979. *Pediatric Oral and Maxillofacial Surgery*. St. Louis: The C.V. Mosby Co.

5. Brook, I., Grimm, S., and Kielich, R.B. 1981. Bacteriology of acute periapical abscess in children. *J. Endodontol.* 7:378–380.

6. Brook, I., Calhoun, L., and Yocum, P. 1981. Beta-lactamase producing isolates of *Bacteroides* species from children. *Antimicrob. Agents Chemother.* 18:164–166.

7. De Leo, A.A., et al. 1974. Incidence of bacteremia following oral prophylaxis on pediatric patients. *Oral Surg.* 37:36–45.

8. Faigel, H.C., and Gaskill, W.F. 1975. Bacteremia in pediatric patients following dental manipulation. *Clin. Pediatr.* 14:562–565.

9. Peterson, L.J., and Peacock, R. 1976. The incidence of bacteremia in pediatric patients following tooth extraction. *Circulation* 53:676–679.

10. Shulman, S.T., et al. 1985. Prevention of bacterial endocarditis. *Am. J. Dis. Child.* 139:232–235.

11. Lindemann, R.A., and Henson, J.L. 1982. The dental management of patients with vascular grafts placed in the treatment of arterial occlusive disease. *J. Am. Dent. Assoc.* 104:625–628.

12. Brooks, S.L. 1980. Survey of compliance with American Heart Association guidelines for prevention of bacterial endocarditis. *J. Am. Dent. Assoc.* 101:41–43.

13. Lampe, R.M., Cheldelin, L.V., and Brown, J. 1978. Brain abscess following dental extraction in a child with cyanotic congenital heart disease. *Pediatrics* 61:659–660.

14. Newman, M.G. 1981. Localized juvenile periodontitis (periodontosis). *Pediatr. Dent.* 3:121–126.

15. Mueller, B.H., et al. 1978. The management of a dental alveolar abscess in an immunosuppressed pancytopenic child. *J. Pedodont.* 3:78–86.

16. Shepherd, J.P. 1978. The management of the oral complications of leukemia. *Oral Surg.* 45:543–548.

17. Casamassimo, P.S. 1982. Renal disease. *In* R.E. Stewart et al. (eds.) *Pediatric Dentistry: Scientific Foundations and Clinical Practice.* St. Louis: The C.V. Mosby Co.

18. Greenberg, M.S., and Cohen, G. 1977. Oral infection in immunosuppressed renal transplant patients. *Oral Surg.* 43:879–885.

19. Kamen, S. 1976. Mental retardation. *In* A.J. Nowak (ed.) *Dentistry for the Handicapped Patient.* St. Louis: The C.V. Mosby Co.

20. Croll, T.P., et al. 1979. Antibiotic prophylaxis for the hydrocephalic dental patient with a shunt. *Pediatr. Dent.* 1:81–85.

21. Moffitt, J.M., et al. 1974. Prediction of tetracycline-induced tooth discoloration. *J. Am. Dent. Assoc.* 88:547–552.

22. Ibsen, K.H., Urist, M.R., and Sognnaes, R.F. 1965. Differences among tetracyclines with respect to the staining of teeth. *J. Pediatr.* 67:459–462.

23. Poliak, S.C., et al. 1985. Minocycline-associated tooth discoloration in young adults. *J. Am. Med. Assoc.* 254:2930–2932.

24. Salman, R.A., et al. 1985. Minocycline induced pigmentation of the oral cavity. *J. Oral Med.* 40:154–157.

CHAPTER 15

Chemotherapeutic Agents in Restorative Dentistry

John A. Sorensen, D.M.D., F.A.C.P.
Perry Klokkevold, D.D.S.

The last decade has witnessed a remarkable increase in the development of chemotherapeutic agents. The creative incorporation and use of these agents in restorative dentistry allows enhanced prosthodontic procedures and improved treatment of maladies arising in prosthodontic patients. This chapter describes how the clinician can use today's chemotherapeutic agents for improvement and long-term maintenance of restorative dentistry. The treatment of microbial infections that develop with prosthodontics will also be discussed.

Fixed prosthodontics

The cornerstone of high-quality fixed prosthodontic treatment that is expediently performed and long lasting is sound periodontal health. Unfortunately, the placement of "esthetic" crowns has been associated with the occurrence of iatrogenic periodontal disease.[1,2] Unsightly gingival inflammation around provisional and permanent crowns usually results from plaque accumulation. With time the plaque matures, resulting in the development of a plaque containing increased numbers of periodontopathic microorganisms.[3] Crowns that are poor fitting, overcontoured, and have a rough surface finish or exposed unglazeable opaque near the margin provide a nidus for plaque development.[3] Gingival health is further compromised when crown margins with these plaque-retaining characteristics are placed subgingivally or are overcontoured.

Fabrication of crowns with excellent marginal adaptation, proper contours, and smooth surfaces should always be placed so that good oral health can be maintained. Effective antimicrobial mouthrinses, used adjunctively, can further limit plaque accumulation, thus enhancing long-term gingival health. Chlorhexidine gluconate mouthrinse (Peridex®) has been shown to be the most effective agent in reducing supragingival plaque and gingivitis when compared to other antimicrobial agents.[4-8]

Gingival enhancement *during* fixed prosthodontics

Gingival bleeding during tooth preparation, gingival retraction, and impression procedures can severely compromise the quality of master stone dies and final crown margin fidelity. Repeated attempts at gingival retraction and impressions because of bleeding within the gingival sulcus are traumatic to the gingival tissues. Subsequent healing may negatively affect the long-term stability and predictability of the gingival margin level in relation to esthetic anterior crown margins.

Recent research using 0.12% chlorhexidine gluconate mouthrinse (Peridex®) to enhance gingival health during fixed prosthodontic procedures has proven highly effective in reducing the plaque index, gingival index, and the number of bleeding sites compared to controls.[9,10] This makes tooth preparation, gingival retraction, and impression procedures easier and more expedient. The frequency of impression remakes in the study was much higher for the control group than in the chlorhexidine rinsing group. An additional finding was that adjunctive chlorhexidine rinsing significantly reduced the numbers of putative periodontal pathogens, retarded bacterial colonization of the subgingival/marginal microflora, and favored the establishment of a microflora compatible with periodontal health.[11,12] The two most common side effects of twice daily rinsing with chlorhexidine are tooth staining and disagreeable or altered taste sensation. Despite these unattractive properties, over 50% of the subjects in the 7-week study noticed a decreased swelling and redness of their gingiva; 92% of the subjects would recommend chlorhexidine rinsing to a friend.[13] Based on the results of this work, diagnostic and treatment regimens are recommended in **Tables 15.1** and **15.2**.

Long-term maintenance of extensive fixed prosthodontics

Patients with extensive fixed prostheses often have periodontally involved abutment teeth with associated gingival recession and exposure of root surfaces. Additionally, dentists frequently place crown margins subgingivally, which results in compromised oral hygiene because of poor access for hygiene measures. These patients are at higher risk for caries and periodontal disease.

Fluorides

As a preventive measure, long-term topical application of fluorides through the vehicle of fluoride stents are often advocated. Fluoride solutions have been shown to be effective in reducing cariogenic plaque,[14,15] and SNF_2 can function as a weak antimicrobial agent against some periodontopathic organisms.[16-18]

Although acidulated phosphate fluorides are effective in reducing cariogenic bacteria, their use in the presence of porcelain restorations is contraindicated. Several studies

---

Table 15.1   Diagnostic and treatment regimen for fixed prosthodontic procedures

---

- Assess gingival health. Determine patient's:

  —oral hygiene abilities
  —plaque levels
  —presence of gingivitis, particularly bleeding on probing
  —pocket depths

- Pocket depths of 4 mm or greater should *first* be treated or referred to a periodontist

- If the patient has bleeding on probing, high plaque levels, or poor oral hygiene, a prophylaxis should be performed and a chlorhexidine regimen initiated at least 2 weeks before tooth preparation and continued for 2 weeks after cementation of the definitive prosthesis (see **Table 15.2**)

- If the patient has minimal plaque levels, good gingival health, and no bleeding on probing, minimal benefit would be achieved with chlorhexidine therapy

---

have demonstrated that acidulated fluorides etch porcelain surfaces, thus removing the glazed surface and resulting in poor esthetics, decreased resistance to staining, and increased plaque accumulation.[19]

A 0.4% stannous fluoride gel applied in a stent will aid in preventing secondary caries around abutment teeth. With a stone cast, a vacuum-made stent can easily be fabricated and will last for several years.

Low-concentration (0.05% NaF_2), over-the-counter fluoride rinses should be recommended for long-term use. Most adults with moderate to extensive restorative or post-periodontal treatment will benefit from long-term low-dose fluoride rinses.

Chlorhexidine

Long-term daily rinsing with chlorhexidine has not been a problem in terms of development of resistant strains of oral microorganisms.[20] With extended (greater than 4 weeks) twice daily usage, significant staining can occur. More frequent prophylaxis to remove stain *before* it becomes a "problem" should be incorporated into the patient's treatment plan.

Many categories of patients are frequently in acrylic resin provisional restorations for an extended period because they have had periodontal treatment, implants (osseointe-gration period and surgical healing), endodontics, or orthodontics. Several factors can significantly reduce staining of provisional restorations when long-term chlorhexidine therapy is desired:

1. To minimize porosity, the acrylic resin provisional restorations should be indirectly fabricated under pressure.

2. The provisional restorations should be well polished with pumice at all aspects,

Table 15.2 Chemotherapeutic agents in restorative dentistry

Purpose	Agent	Regimen	Instructions
Gingival enhancement in fixed prosthodontics	0.12% chlorhexidine gluconate (Peridex)	15 mL bid 30 s rinse; start 2 weeks before tooth preparation, continue for 2 weeks after final cementation	Brush and floss teeth first. Rinse with chlorhexidine 15 mL bid for 30 s and expectorate; do not rinse, eat, or drink for 30 min
Long-term maintenance of extensive fixed prosthodontics	0.4% stannous fluoride gel/ over-the-counter sodium fluoride rinses	Fluoride gel placed in stent/daily rinsing	Once a day place gel in stents, hold both maxillary and mandibular stents in mouth for 4 min; expectorate excess gel; do not rinse, eat, or drink for 30 min
Long-term maintenance of periodontal-prostheses	0.12% chlorhexidine gluconate (Peridex)	Apply with interproximal brush or dilute 3:1 for irrigation device once daily	Apply with interproximal brush or irrigation device
Denture stomatitis (candidiasis)	Nystatin pastilles	400,000–600,000 units qid, continue for 48 h after symptoms have resolved	Suck on pastilles until completely dissolved qid. Continue for 48 h after symptoms have resolved
Denture stomatitis (candidiasis)	Ketoconazole	200–400 mg/d	200–400 mg/d
Severe denture stomatitis (candidiasis)	Consult with patient's physician on therapeutic options		
Recurrent herpes labialis	Topical acyclovir (Zovirax, 5% ointment)	Apply as needed to affected areas	Apply 5% ointment as needed to affected areas
Systemic herpes infection (herpes simplex virus)	Acyclovir (Zovirax)	IV 250 mg/m² q8h for 7 d	IV 250 mg/m² q8h for 7 d
		Oral 200–400 mg 5 times/d for 7–10 d	Oral 200–400 mg 5 times/d for 7–10 d

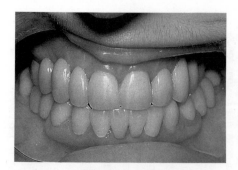 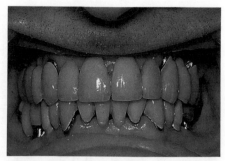

Fig 15.1   A patient who has been in acrylic resin provisional restorations for 4 months. There is only minimal staining because of the twice daily rinses with chlorhexidine.

Fig 15.2   This patient has been applying chlorhexidine, via a small interproximal brush, for over 4 years. Staining has been minimal.

including the gingival margin area, interproximals surfaces, and gingival embrasures of fixed partial dentures.

Figure 15.1 shows a patient who has been in acrylic resin provisional restorations for 4 months while awaiting osseointegration of maxillary implant fixtures. The patient has been rinsing twice daily with chlorhexidine and has minimal staining.

For patients with periodontal prostheses, an alternative method of delivering chlorhexidine can be used to minimize staining. One method employs dipping a small interproximal brush, such as the Proxabrush® in chlorhexidine during daily oral hygiene measures. **Figure 15.2** shows a patient who has been using this method of application for over 4 years with great benefit to gingival health; the patient has had minimal staining.

Sulcular irrigation may increase the effectiveness of chlorhexidine (see chapter 11) in the subgingival area, but it is unclear whether or not there is a decrease in stain.

Removable prosthodontics—candidiasis

Tissues covered by removable prostheses are at risk of becoming irritated, inflamed, and possibly infected if oral hygiene is poor and/or host resistance is diminished. Denture stomatitis (inflammation of oral mucosal tissues adjacent to dentures) can be limited to a localized area of erythema under an appliance or it can be associated with generalized inflammation. Plaque and denudation can sometimes be seen throughout the mouth.

Plaque and debris resulting from poor oral hygiene accumulates on denture surfaces in a manner similar to that on natural teeth of dentate patients. However, rougher surfaces and porosities in denture acrylic resin facilitate retention of microorganisms. Thus, tissues in contact with denture surfaces are constantly exposed to and irritated by bacterial and fungal toxins as well as the rough surfaces themselves. Oral tissues that are covered for extended periods of time may be inhabited by different microorganisms than are noncovered tissues. More virulent microbes may be selected and may potentiate denture stomatitis. See chapter 10 for a discussion of adverse microbiological effects.

Candida albicans is a frequent organism to opportunistically dominate the microenvironment under a denture. Candidiasis is typically seen as whitish plaques that can be removed. The underlying tissue is very red and painful. Denture stomatitis is commonly caused by *C. albicans*, but other species may cause or contribute to it.

Diagnosis

Candida species are yeast-like fungi that are described as opportunistic because they only cause infections when conditions are optimal. They are frequently present, in small numbers, in the normal oral microflora. A method to determine the presence of a candidal infection is to examine affected tissue under a microscope. *C. albicans* appears as a fine, branching, nonsegmented mycelial net, sometimes with small, oval, budding, thin-walled cells and clusters of microspores.[21] When a diagnosis of candidiasis is confirmed, all contributory factors, local and systemic, should be examined. *Candida* frequently becomes infective when host resistance is lowered during antibiotic treatment (see chapter 10), nutritional deficiency, or immunosuppressive therapy (see chapter 18).

Treatment

Clean, smooth prosthetic surfaces are more resistant to plaque and debris accumulation and retention than porous surfaces. Thus, it is imperative to replace or reline rough, porous denture surfaces and to professionally clean appliances when infections occur. Having the patient not wear the infected dentures as much as possible will also aid recovery.

Minor cases of denture stomatitis may respond well to cleaning and polishing of prostheses and improved oral hygiene. More extensive cases of stomatitis may require antimicrobial therapy to be resolved. Nystatin and ketoconazole are useful in treating oral candidiasis. The authors' experience is that nystatin is most effective and ketoconazole is quite expensive. More resistant infections will require treatment with amphotericin B, and discussion with a specialist and/or the patient's physician is recommended. Twice daily mouthrinsing with chlorhexidine gluconate, which has been shown to be effective against fungal organisms, should also be considered (see chapter 8).

All measures that enhance the patient's overall general health are useful in treating candidiasis. Consider recommendations to improve nutrition and good oral hygiene habits. It is also important to discontinue any antibiotic therapy, if possible, because this may have precipitated the candidal infection. Consult and work with the patient's physician when more than minor host-related conditions contribute to the problem.

Recurrent herpes precipitated by restorative dental treatment

Prolonged restorative dental procedures often place stress on oral and perioral soft tissues. In patients with a history of recurrent herpetic infections, stress induced by dental procedures may precipitate a herpetic episode.

Primary oral infection with herpes simplex virus often results in acute herpetic gingivostomatitis, which is actually a systemic infection with oral lesions. This usually occurs in young individuals, but it can and does occur in adults. The virus enters the body through the oral mucosa and causes an acute illness. The patient becomes febrile with cervical lymphadenopathy. Vesicles form on the mucosa, rupture, and result in ulcerations with erythematous halos. The gingivae are hypertrophic, bright red, and painful. After 10 to 14 days the acute symptoms subside, but the causative virus is not eliminated. It apparently remains latent in the nerve ganglia, supplying the site of initial infection.

Recurrent lesions initially form blisters (common cold sore or fever blister) with clear serous fluid. They rupture to form ulcerations, which resolve in about 10 to 14 days. Many factors are associated with recurrent herpes infections. Among them are respiratory infections, sunlight exposure, fever, trauma, exposure to chemicals, and emotional stress. Dental procedures can cause significant emotional and physiological stress as well as local trauma and thus often precipitate herpes lesions.

Diagnosis

Recurrent infections with herpes virus are often diagnosed on the basis of history and clinical experience. Herpes simplex virus can be isolated from early lesions and diagnosed by tissue culture. However, it takes several days for laboratory test results. Various tests (immunologic and serologic) are useful in the diagnosis, but they are technique sensitive and/or have limitations.

Treatment

Most strains of herpes virus are susceptible to 5-iodo-2'-deoxuridine and other nucleo-side analogs. Topical application of Zovirax® is useful in decreasing the spread and severity of the recurrent infection. Local application of antibiotics is sometimes advised to prevent superinfection of ulcerations. For symptomatic relief, especially before meals, local anesthetics can be applied to affected areas. In patients with a previous history of herpes infection secondary to dental procedures, pretreatment with Zovirax® may reduce the severity of infection.

Summary

Future developments in chemotherapeutic agents are sure to offer new and innovative ways to enhance restorative dental procedures. Present antimicrobial mouthrinses can enhance gingival health to make fixed prosthodontic procedures easier and more expedient. These mouthrinses also improve the tissue/restoration interface for long-term maintenance of extensive fixed prosthodontics. Available chemotherapeutic agents can control ailments such as denture stomatitis or herpetic eruptions that may arise from extended restorative dental procedures.

References

1. Löe, H. 1968. Reactions of marginal periodontal tissues to restorative procedures. *Int. Dent. J.* 18:759–778.

2. Silness, J. 1970. Periodontal conditions in patients treated with dental bridges. II. The influence of full and partial crowns on plaque accumulation, development of gingivitis and pocket formation. *J. Periodont. Res.* 5:219–224.

3. Sorensen, J.A. 1989. A rationale for comparison of plaque-retaining properties of crown systems. *J. Prosthet. Dent.* 62:264–269.

4. Wennstrom, J., and Lindhe, J. 1986. The effect of mouthrinses on parameters characterizing human periodontal disease. *J. Clin. Periodontol.* 13:86–93.

5. Segreto, V.A., Collins, E.M., Beiswagner, B.B., dela Rosa, M., Isaucs, R.C., Lang, N.P., Mallat, M.E., and Meckel, A.H. 1986. A comparison of mouthrinses containing two concentrations of chlorhexidine. *J. Periodont. Res.* Suppl:23–32.

6. Siegrist, A.E., Gusberti, F.A., Brecx, M.L., Weber, H.P., and Lang, N.P. 1986. Efficacy of supervised rinsing with chlorhexidine digluconate in comparison to phenolic and plant alkaloid compounds. *J. Periodont. Res.* Suppl:60–73.

7. Gusberti, F.A., Sampathkumar, P., Siegrist, B.E., and Lang, N.P. 1988. Microbiological and clinical effects of chlorhexidine gluconate and hydrogen peroxide mouthrinses on developing plaque and gingivitis. *J. Periodontol.* 15:60–67.

8. Svatun, B., Gjermo, P., Eriksen, H.M., and Rolla, G. 1977. A comparison of the plaque-inhibiting effect of stannous fluoride and chlorhexidine. *Acta Odontol. Scand.* 35:247–250.

9. Sorensen, J.A., Flemmig, T.F., Doherty, F.M., Newman, M.G. 1988. Gingival enhancement in fixed prosthodontics. I. Clinical findings. *J. Dent. Res.* 67:374 (Abstr. no. 2091).

10. Sorensen, J.A., Flemmig, T.F., Doherty, F.M., Newman, M.G., and Lee, J.J. (Submitted.) Gingival enhancement in fixed prosthodontics. I. Clinical findings. *J. Prosthet. Dent.*

11. Flemmig, T.F., Sorensen, J.A., Newman, M.G., Nachnani, S., Calsina, G., and Doherty, F.M. 1988. Gingival enhancement in fixed prosthodontics. II. Microbiologic findings. *J. Dent. Res.* 67:374 (Abstr. no. 2092).

12. Sorensen, J.A., Flemmig, T.F., Newman, M.G., Nachnani, S., Calsina, G., and Doherty, F.M. (Submitted.) Gingival enhancement in fixed prosthodontics. II. Microbiologic findings. *J. Prosthet. Dent.*

13. Sorensen, J.A., Flemmig, T.F., and Newman, M.G. (Submitted.) Gingival enhancement in fixed prosthodontics. III. Properties of chlorhexidine gluconate and patient questionnaire. *J. Prosthet. Dent.*

14. Andres, C.J., Shaffer, J.C., and Windeler, A.S., Jr. 1974. Comparisons of antibacterial properties of stannous fluoride and sodium fluoride mouthwashes. *J. Dent. Res.* 53:457–460.

15. Gross, A., and Tinanoff, N. 1977. Effect of SnF$_2$ mouthrinse on initial bacterial colonization of tooth enamel. *J. Dent. Res.* 56:1179–1183.

16. Loesche, W.J. 1976. Chemotherapy of dental plaque infections. *Oral Sci. Rev.* 9:65–107.

17. Yoon, N.A., and Berry, C.W. 1979. The antimicrobial effect of fluorides (acidulated phosphate, sodium and stannous) on *Actinomyces viscosus. J. Dent. Res.* 58:1824–1829.

18. Mazza, J., Newman, M.G., and Sims, T.N. 1981. Clinical and antimicrobial effect of stannous fluoride on periodontitis. *J. Clin. Periodontol.* 8:203–212.

19. Copps, D.P., Lacy, A.M., Curtis, T., and Carman, J.E. 1984. Effects of topical fluorides on five low-fusing dental porcelains. *J. Prosthet. Dent.* 52:340–343.

20. Briner, W.W., Grossman, E., Bucker, R.Y., Rebitski, G.F., Sox, T.E., Setser, R.E., and Ebert, M.C. 1986. Effect of chlorhexidine gluconate mouthrinse on plaque bacterial. *J. Periodont. Res.* Suppl:44–52.

21. Schuster, G. 1983. *Oral Microbiology and Infectious Disease.* Baltimore, Md.: Williams and Wilkins.

CHAPTER 16

Antimicrobials in Implant Dentistry

Thomas F. Flemmig, Dr. med. dent.
Michael G. Newman, D.D.S.

Rationale

Although various forms of dental implants have been used for over 20 years, the use of endosseous implants has rapidly become a major therapeutic modality.[1] With a higher number of implants being placed and with improved longevity, the frequency of implant complications is expected to rise. Implant complications can occur during fixture placement and in the early healing phases after surgery. Some problems can occur after uncovering of implants and abutment placement as well as during the maintenance phase of treatment (see **Table 16.1**).

Intraoperative complications are mainly technique and/or system related and include injury of anatomic structures, excessive bleeding, and failure to achieve primary implant stability. Early *postoperative* complications include infection, excessive bleeding, flap dehiscence, and failure to achieve osseointegration. *Peri-implant complications* occur during implant maintenance and can be classified into *(1)* compromised success, *(2)* failing implant, and *(3)* failed implant. Different forms of peri-implant infections are associated with elevated levels of specific microorganisms that appear to play an etiologic role in the associated infection[2-20] (see **Table 16.2**).

The subgingival microflora found in a healthy peri-implant environment is similar to the subgingival flora of periodontally healthy teeth; correspondingly, the microflora found in peri-implant disease is similar to that found in periodontal disease.[10] Other implicated etiological factors of peri-implant complications are occlusal overload and systemic diseases.

To date, little pertinent information is available to guide the prevention and treatment of implant complications. The available modalities for infectious implant complications can only be extrapolated from research results in periodontology and oral surgery and brought into perspective with the current knowledge of implant dentistry. In this chapter the presently available information is compiled to give suggestions for the

---

Table 16.1   Implant complications (incidence)[2,3,39,53,64]

Implant placement and uncovering

Intraoperative

- Injury of anatomical structures
- Excessive bleeding
- No primary stability

Postoperative

- Infection
- Excessive bleeding
- Flap dehiscence (<5%†)
- No osseointegration

Peri-implant complications during maintenance

- Compromised success
  —gingivitis (8%–44%, increasing with time)
  —gingival hyperplasia (1%–7%)
  —fistula (<1.5%)
  —implant fracture
- Failing implant
  —progressing vertical bone loss, but still in function (5%*)
- Failed implant
  —failure within first year (3%–7%)
  —failure after the first year (1%–13% increasing with time)

---

*Derived figure.
†(Incidence).

prevention and *management* of infectious implant complications in the postoperative phase and during implant maintenance. The information in this text is mainly relevant to endosseous implants because their use prevails and appears to outweigh other implant types. However, most of the principles described here may also apply to subperiosteal and transosteal implants.

Implant surgery

Placement surgery

Placement of dental implants (fixtures) involves the jawbones and the overlying soft tissues. Implant therapy is usually performed on an outpatient basis and can be compared to oral surgical or periodontal procedures involving the same tissues. Aseptic and sterile techniques, including disinfecting the surgical field with chlorhexidine or

Table 16.2   Microorganisms associated with peri-implant complications[2-12]

- *Staphylococcus* sp.
- *Actinomyces* sp.
- Surface translocating bacteria (STB)
- *Wolinella* sp.
- *Capnocytophaga*
- Black-pigmented *Bacteroides* sp.
  — *Bacteroides intermedius*
  — *Bacteroides gingivalis*
- *Fusobacterium* sp.
- *Entamoeba gingivalis*
- Motile rods
- Fusiforms
- Spirochetes
- Enteric gram-negative bacteria
- *Candida albicans*

iodine, is recommended.[21] Under these conditions the incidence of postoperative wound infections after regular oral surgical or periodontal procedures is low and does not usually require perioperative antibiotics.[22-25] In general, a prophylactic regimen is medically and economically warranted if the incidence of the complication to be prevented is high and/or is associated with severe sequellae. The incidence of postoperative wound infections after implant placement and uncovering has not been assessed. Hence, at this point the benefit of any prophylactic antibiotic regimen in implant surgery is questionable and needs to be determined.

When a specific surgical protocol is followed that includes perioperative antibiotics, one should adhere to these guidelines. It is possible, although unlikely, that the antibiotic regimen has an impact on the success of the specific implant system. The surgical protocols of the implant systems available in North America and Europe do not equivocally recommend routine prophylactic perioperative systemic antibiotics.[21,26-30] In general, prophylactic antibiotics to reduce the incidence of postoperative infections are indicated when *(1)* the patient's host response is reduced; *(2)* a massive bacterial contamination of noncontaminated tissues is expected (i.e., surgery in inflamed sites; or *(3)* an extensive procedure and/or large volumes of foreign material threaten to overwhelm the ability of the host to defend itself.[31] If the expected time of surgery exceeds 2 hours, the incidence of postoperative complications increases.[32] Only in these circumstances do systemic antibiotics seem to be warranted when using an implant system that does not follow a protocol including routine perioperative antibiotics.[33]

Another indication for systemic antibiotics may be the immediate insertion of implants after traumatic tooth loss where contamination is expected.[29] However, if antibiotics are given for prophylaxis of postoperative wound infection, **it is imperative to administer the first dose preoperatively** (for penicillin V 2g per os, 1 hour preoperatively).[34,35] The duration of most antibiotic regimens for implant placement surgery extends over 3 to 10 days.[21,26] However, it has been demonstrated that prolongation of prophylaxis beyond the first 3 postoperative days may not provide additional protection.[33,36-38]

For some implant systems, topical antibiotics (e.g., bacitracin and tetracycline) are recommended to be placed into the hole for the cover screw during implant placement.[26] There is little scientific evidence for the benefit of this regimen but the risk is low and such treatment does not appear to cause harm.

The same considerations regarding systemic antibiotics apply for one- and two-stage systems. A one-stage implant is immediately exposed to the oral environment and bacterial colonization begins during the crucial bone healing phase. During this time it is imperative to prevent loading of the implant in order to allow osseointegration to occur. In most cases a health-associated flora colonizes one-stage implants immediately after insertion. However, in cases of early failure, bacteria associated with peri-implant complications were found.[6,11] It appears prudent to aid oral hygiene with adjunctive antimicrobial rinsing (e.g., 15 mL of 0.12% chlorhexidine gluconate [Peridex®] q12h) during the time of bone healing for as much as 3 to 6 months to prevent bacterial colonization (see **Table 16.3**).

If patients with immunodeficiencies, metabolic diseases, risks for metastatic infections secondary to transient bacteremia, or irradiation in the head and neck area are selected for implant insertion, the same principles for prophylactic antibiotic coverage apply as for other oral surgical and periodontal procedures (see chapters 13, 17, and 18).

Stage-two surgery

The second-stage surgery or *uncovering* of the implant and placement of the abutment involves mainly soft tissues. Peri-implant pocket probing depth is initially determined by the thickness of the peri-implant mucosa, and mucosal flap thinning during the uncovering stage can initially prevent deep peri-implant pockets.[39] Existing keratinized gingiva should be preserved by splitting it into two halves and placing one part on the buccal and the other on the lingual side of the implant.[40]

Analogous to periodontal flap surgery, rinsing with 15 mL of 0.12% chlorhexidine every 12 hours may reduce plaque accumulation, enhance gingival health, and improve healing.[41-43] The epithelial and HeLa cell growth inhibition of chlorhexidine found in vitro[44,45] does not seem to have any clinical effect on wound healing after mucoperiosteal surgery[41-43] (see **Table 16.3**).

Table 16.3 Antimicrobial regimens in implant surgery and implant maintenance

---

	Topical	*Systemic*
Implant surgery		
Placement surgery Preoperative:	• 0.12% chlorhexidine rinse *or* • 2% iodine (immediately preoperatively)	• According to surgical protocol of implant system *or* If surgery > 2 h or is extensive: —penicillin V* 2 g PO (1 h preoperatively)
Postoperatively:	One-stage systems only: • 0.12% chlorhexidine 15 mL q12h 3–6 mo	• According to surgical protocol of implant system *or* If surgery > 2 h or is extensive: —penicillin V* 500 mg q6h PO 1 d
Uncovering surgery (two-stage systems only)		
Postoperatively:	• 0.12% chlorhexidine 15 mL q12h for 6 wk	None
Implant maintenance	• Oral hygiene instruction/reinforcement • Maintenance (plastic scaler & rubber cup) every 3 mo or customized	None

*Amoxicillin or Augmentin may also be administered, depending on individual circumstances and clinical judgment.

Prophylactic systemic antibiotics at this stage are only necessary in medically compromised patients, and the general prophylactic principles apply (see chapter 17).

Implant maintenance

Oral hygiene instruction is of paramount importance for patients treated with implants. Individual needs should be reinforced and updated regularly at each and every maintenance visit. Oral hygiene must be adjusted to the specific anatomical situation for each individual patient using manual toothbrush, rotary electric toothbrush,[46,47] floss, toothpick, and subgingival and/or supragingival irrigation with water or medicament. Special implant cleaning devices such as Postcare® are also available.

Implant maintenance should include supragingival and subgingival debridement with a specially designed plastic scaler, Perioaid®, Superfloss®, Postcare, and/or rubber cup polishing. Instruments that may injure the implant and abutment surface, such as stainless steel curettes, should be avoided because a rough surface may enhance bacterial adhesion.

In partially edentulous patients, a 3-month maintenance regimen has been shown to maintain peri-implant health and to prevent subgingival colonization of microorganisms associated with peri-implant complications.[48,49] In partially edentulous patients the recall interval is often determined by the remaining natural dentition. In fully edentulous patients one should follow the same regimen and, if necessary, customize the recall to the patient's needs (see **Table 16.3**).

Treatment of implant complications

Treatment of postoperative implant complications

After implant fixture placement   *Acute postoperative infections* usually occur on the third or fourth day after surgery.[50] Surgical drainage should be established immediately and a culture taken for antibiotic susceptibility testing. At the same time, empiric antibiotic therapy with penicillin V, amoxicillin, or Augmentin® per os should be initiated. In case of penicillin allergy, erythromycin, metronidazole, or clindamycin can be given alternatively.[51] The antibiotics should be administered 3 days beyond the occurrence of marked clinical improvement (usually at the fourth day), hence for a minimum of 7 days. The patient must be monitored very closely. If within the first 2 days no clinical improvement occurs, the antibiotic should be changed according to the susceptibility test results. If no improvement after specific systemic antibiotic therapy occurs, one should consider removing the implants. In serious cases of fulminant and spreading infections, the patient may need to be admitted to a hospital for high-dose intravenous specific antibiotic treatment. The survival of an implant in cases of early infection is always questionable.

If *flap dehiscences* over the implant occur during the healing phase (3 to 6 months postoperatively) one should eliminate the possible causes (e.g., pressure of denture on the implant) and eventually excise the soft tissue around the dehiscence. Whether flap coverage should be attempted or the implant left exposed is controversial.[52] Recently, attempts to regenerate osseous tissue in areas of dehiscence using barrier techniques such as Gore-Tex® have suggested that this approach may prove to be efficacious. Topical antimicrobials should be given to prevent plaque accumulation in cases where the implant is left exposed. These may be administered by rinse or irrigation.

The first evaluation of the clinical signs of osseointegration are usually assessed during the stage-two surgery or during the time when a one-stage implant should be

---

Table 16.4   Treatment of postoperative implant complications

---

After implant placement

Wound infection
- Drainage
- Antibiotic susceptibility testing
- Penicillin* 500 mg q6h for ≥ 7 d
- If no improvement within 2 d:
    —change antibiotic according to susceptibility test results
    or
    —remove implant
- In fulminant cases:
    —admit to hospital for IV antibiotic therapy

Flap dehiscence
- Eliminate cause
- Excise tissue around dehiscence
- If implant is exposed:
    —0.12% chlorhexidine 15 mL q12h

No primary osseointegration
- Remove implant

After uncovering implants (two-stage systems only)

Wound infection
- Mechanical debridement and
- 0.12% chlorhexidine rinse
- If fluctuance:
    —drainage
    —antibiotic susceptibility testing
    —penicillin* 500 mg q6h for ≥ 7 d
- If no improvement within 2 d:
    —change antibiotic according to susceptibility test results
- If implant is mobile, remove it
- In fulminant cases:
    —admit to hospital for IV antibiotic therapy

---

*Amoxicillin or Augmentin may also be administered, depending on individual circumstances and clinical judgment.

loaded. If the clinical signs indicate that *osseointegration has not occurred*, the implant, including the connective tissue lining of the socket, should be removed. Some authors suggest that it may be possible to insert another implant at the same site using barrier techniques, bone grafting materials, or combinations of these approaches. At the present time these techniques are evolving and no definitive recommendation can be made. Thus, it may be prudent to wait for bone healing to take place before inserting a new implant (see **Table 16.4**).

After uncovering of implants (two-stage systems only)   Acute infections after stage-two (uncovering) surgery are rare and should be treated with debridement and local antimicrobials. If fluctuance is present, drainage should be established and systemic antibiotics given. The drugs of first choice are penicillin, amoxicillin, or Augmentin. If no clinical improvement occurs within the first 24 hours, culture and antibiotic susceptibility testing should be performed, followed by specific systemic antibiotics. Mobile implants should be removed (see **Table 16.4**).

Treatment of peri-implant complications during maintenance

Peri-implant gingivitis   The incidence of *peri-implant gingivitis* increases with time and, similar to natural teeth, is associated with increased plaque accumulation.[3,53] *It should be treated by removal of the cause: plaque.* Oral hygiene adapted to the specific anatomic situation should be given, regular professional cleanings initiated, and the recall interval shortened. Adjunctive to mechanical home care, the use of antimicrobial rinses[54,55] and supragingival or subgingival irrigation with antimicrobials or water may be beneficial. In several studies on natural teeth,[56-58] naturally occurring gingivitis was reduced most by a regimen of adjunctive supragingival irrigation with 300 mL of water, followed by irrigation with 200 mL of 0.06% chlorhexidine. Both a 0.12% chlorhexidine rinse (15 mL twice a day) and once daily 500-mL water irrigation also significantly reduced gingivitis, but to a lesser extent. However, supragingival irrigation with water had only limited effect beyond brushing on supragingival and subgingival plaque. These findings in natural teeth may be extrapolated and help determine the most efficacious treatment for peri-implant gingivitis. It is noteworthy that most topical antimicrobials are only effective during the time of application.[59] An exception is chlorhexidine, which may be effective up to 8 hours because of its substantivity (see chapter 8). If after a course of antimicrobial treatment the patient cannot maintain peri-implant health, the treatment may be repeated and prolonged. However, despite the safety of some antimicrobial agents in long-term use, their side effects (e.g., staining and taste alteration) may be a nuisance. Hence, in patients treated with implants, supragingival irrigation with water or use of adjunctive mechanical devices may be a beneficial long-term oral hygiene adjunct without significant side effects.

If peri-implant gingivitis is refractory to mechanical and antimicrobial therapy and is associated with deep probing depths, pocket elimination surgery may help to improve peri-implant health. A positive correlation has been found between pocket probing depth and gingivitis severity.[3,16] However, it is unclear if deep peri-implant pockets alone reduce implant longevity. Gingival extension surgery to ease oral hygiene may be indicated in cases of persistent gingivitis associated with lack of keratinized and/or attached gingiva, although most of the studies did not find a positive correlation between the width of attached/keratinized gingiva and peri-implant health.[14,16,60]

Gingival hyperplasia   This is a rare peri-implant complication and may result from bacterial plaque and/or insufficient space between the implant prosthesis and peri-implant mucosa. Improperly seated implant components may also lead to peri-implant gingival hyperplasia. Mechanical debridement followed by a home care regimen with adjunctive irrigating or rinsing with antimicrobials, as described for the treatment of peri-implant gingivitis, should be attempted first. If the prosthesis design does not permit proper oral hygiene, the prosthesis should be temporarily removed or a provisional restoration with wide-open embrasures made. After the lesion has resolved, a new restoration should be manufactured that permits better oral hygiene. In refractory cases, a susceptibility test of the putative pathogenic plaque bacteria should be performed and specific systemic antibiotics administered. In some cases, pocket elimination surgery or gingivectomy, followed by a stringent maintenance regimen, may resolve the lesion (see **Table 16.5**).

Peri-implant fistula The occurrence of a peri-implant fistula should be treated by excision and mechanical debridement.[51] Antimicrobials and specific antibiotics may be given in refractory cases after susceptibility testing of the subgingival plaque. One should also check the proper seat of all implant components.

Failing implants Implants that are failing *progressively* lose marginal bone. Treatment should be aimed toward eliminating all possible etiological factors such as

---

Table 16.5 Treatment of peri-implant complications during maintenance

Mechanical/surgical	*Antimicrobials*
Gingivitis	
• Oral hygiene instruction/reinforcement	• Adjunctive
• Mechanical debridement (plastic scaler & rubber cup)	—water 300 mL & 0.06% chlorhexidine 200 mL supragingival irrigation q24h
• Shorter maintenance intervals If insufficient space between mucosa & denture, remove denture If refractory and associated with deep pocket and/or lack of keratinized gingiva: —pocket elimination *and/or* —gingiva extension	*or* —0.12% chlorhexidine rinse 15 mL q12h *or* —water 500 mL supragingival irrigation q24h
Gingival hyperplasia	
• Oral hygiene instruction/reinforcement	• Adjunctive —water 300 mL & 0.06% chlorhexidine 200 mL supragingival irrigation q24h
• Mechanical debridement (plastic scaler & rubber cup)	*or*
• Shorter maintenance intervals	—0.12% chlorhexidine rinse 15 mL q12h
• Check seat of implant components If insufficient space between mucosa & denture, remove denture and redesign If refractory, perform pocket elimination surgery or gingivectomy	*or* —water 500 mL supragingival irrigation q24h • If refractory —susceptibility test and specific systemic antibiotics

Table 16.5 continues

Table 16.5   continued

Mechanical/surgical	Antimicrobials
Fistula	
• Oral hygiene instruction/reinforcement • Mechanical debridement (plastic scaler & rubber cup) • Excision • Check seat of implant components	• Adjunctive —water 300 mL & 0.06% chlorhexidine 200 mL supragingival irrigation q24h *or* —0.12% chlorhexidine rinse 15 mL q12h • If refractory —susceptibility test and specific systemic antibiotics
Failing implant	
• Oral hygiene instruction/reinforcement • Mechanical debridement (plastic scaler & rubber cup) • Shorter maintenance intervals If refractory and associated with deep pocket and/or lack of keratinized gingiva: —pocket elimination with or without gingiva extension —regenerative surgery	• Adjunctive —water 300 mL & 0.06% chlorhexidine 200 mL supragingival irrigation q24h *or* —0.12% chlorhexidine rinse 15 mL q12h • If refractory —susceptibility test and specific systemic antibiotics
Failed implant	
• Implant removal	

occlusal overload and bacterial/fungal infection. Therapeutic principles for periodontal disease in natural teeth are often applied in failing implants despite little proof that this extrapolation is valid. According to some reports, "periodontal" surgery in failing implants could improve peri-implant health over a short observation period.[61] Regenerative techniques used in periodontics may be another way to treat failing implants.[62] Adjunctive irrigation or rinsing with antimicrobials as described for the treatment of peri-implant gingivitis should also be initiated. The subgingival microflora of failing implants can be associated with periodontal pathogens, non-oral pathogens, and *Candida albicans*.[9] Hence, appropriate microbiological analyses and antibiotic susceptibility testing should precede any antibiotic therapy.

If susceptibility testing is not available or if therapy should start before the test results are available, the antibiotics most likely to be effective against putative pathogenic bacteria in peri-implant complications appear to be tetracycline, penicillin, amoxicillin, Augmentin, and metronidazole. Analogous to periodontal disease, one course of systemic tetracycline has the potential to eliminate bacteria associated with peri-implant complications.[63] However, because nonspecific antibiotic treatment may select for resistant strains and result in fungal overgrowth, antibiotic susceptibility testing should always be attempted in the treatment of failing implants refractory to mechanical and topical antimicrobial therapy (see **Table 16.5**). *Whenever systemic antibiotics are administered, concomitant topical plaque control agents are always recommended.*

Failed implants Implants that have lost bony support and do not serve their function should be removed early to prevent further bone loss (see **Table 16.5**).

For all the antimicrobials recommended above, it is imperative to rule out allergies and interferences with other drugs the patient is taking. If necessary, alternative drugs need to be administered.

In implant dentistry the indications for antimicrobial therapy are still vague and mostly empirical. Further investigations regarding the management of peri-implant complications must determine the optimal therapy for the various peri-implant complications.

References

1. Worthington, P. 1988. Current implant use. *J. Dent. Educ.* 12:692–695.

2. Lekholm, U., Ericsson, I., Adell, R., and Slots, J. 1986. The condition of the soft tissues at tooth and fixture abutments supporting fixed bridges. A microbiological and histological study. *J. Clin. Periodontol.* 13:558–562.

3. Lekholm, U., Adell, R., Lindhe, J., Brånemark, P.-I., Ericsson, B., Rocker, B., Lindvall, A.-M., and Yoneyma, T. 1986. Marginal tissue reactions at osseointegrated titanium fixtures. II. A cross-sectional retrospective study. *Int. J. Oral Surg.* 15:53–61.

4. Rams, T.E., Roberts, T.W., Tatum, H., Jr., and Keyes, P.H. 1984. The subgingival microflora associated with human dental implants. *J. Prosthet. Dent.* 51:529–534.

5. Rams, T.E., and Link, C.C., Jr. 1983. Microbiology of failing dental implants in humans: electron microscopic observations. *J. Oral Implantol.* 11:93–100.

6. Mombelli, A., Buser, D., and Lang, N.P. 1988. Colonization of osseointegrated implants in edentulous patients. *J. Dent. Res.* 67:287 (Abstr. no. 1394).

7. Mombelli, A., Van Oosten, M.A.C., Schürch, E., and Lang, N.P. 1987. The microbiota associated with successful or failing osseointegrated titanium implants. *Oral Microbiol. Immunol.* 2:145–151.

8. Krekeler, G., Pelz, K., and Nelissen, R. 1986. Mikrobielle Besiedlung der Zahnfleischtaschen am künstlichen Titanpfeiler. *Dtsch. Zahnärztl. Z.* 41:569–572.

9. Alcoforado, G.A.P., Feik, D., Rams, T.E., Rosenberg, E., and Slots, J. 1989. Microbiology of failing osseointegrated dental implants. *Abstr. Am. Soc. Microbiol.* 457 (Abstr. no. C 382).

10. Sanz, M., Newman, M.G., Nachnani, S., Holt, R., Stewart, R., and Flemmig, T. (In press, 1990.) Characterization of the subgingival microbial flora around endosteal sapphire dental implants in partially edentulous patients. *Int. J. Maxillofac. Implants.*

11. Nakou, M., Mikx, F.H., Oosterwaal, P.J.M., and Kruijsen, J.C.W.M. 1987. Early microbial colonisation of permucosal implants in edentulous patients. *J. Dent. Res.* 66:1654–1657.

12. Holt, R., Newman, M.G., Kratochvil, F., Jeswani, S., Bugler, M., Khorsandi, S., and Sanz, M. 1986. The clinical and microbial characterization of peri-implant environment. *J. Dent. Res.* 65:247 (Abstr. no. 703).

13. Brandes, R., Beamer, B., Holt, S.C., Kornman, K., and Lang, N.P. 1988. Clinical-microscopic observation of ligature induced "peri-implantitis" around osseointegrated implants. *J. Dent. Res.* 67:287 (Abstr. no. 1397).

14. Strub, J.R., Garberthüel, T. W., and Schärer, P. 1988. Role of attached gingiva for peri-implant health in dogs. *J. Dent. Res.* 67:287 (Abstr. no. 1396).

15. Koth, D.L., McKinney, R.V., and Steflik, D.E. 1987. Microscopic study of the hygiene effect on peri-implant gingival tissue. *J. Dent. Res.* 66:186 (Abstr. no. 639).

16. Flemmig, T.F., and Höltje, W.-J. 1988. Periimplantäre Mukosa und Knochen bei Titan-Implantaten: Die Rolle von Plaque, Zahnstein, befestigter Gingiva und Suprakonstruktion. *Z. Zahnärztl. Implantol.* 4:153–157.

17. Zarb, G.A., and Symington, J.M. 1983. Osseointegrated dental implants: Preliminary report on a replication study. *J. Prosthet. Dent.* 50:271–276.

18. Spörlein, E., and Stein, R. 1987. Nachuntersuchung von 100 Tübinger Sofortimplantaten unter Berücksichtigung der parodontalen Situation, der Belastung und der knöchernen Integration. *Z. Zahnärztl. Implantol.* 3:13–17.

19. Bergman, B. 1983. Evaluation of the results of treatment with osseointegrated implants by the Swedish National Board of Health and Welfare. *J. Prosthet. Dent.* 50:114–115.

20. Lindquist, L.W., Rockler, B., and Carlsson, G.E. 1988. Bone resorption around fixtures in edentulous patients treated wtih mandibular fixed tissue-integrated prostheses. *J. Prosthet. Dent.* 59:59–63.

21. Adell, R., Lekholm, U., and Brånemark, P.-I. 1985. Surgical procedures. *In* P.-I. Brånemark, G.A. Zarb, and T. Albrektsson (eds.) *Tissue-Integrated Prostheses. Osseointegration in Clinical Dentistry.* Chicago: Quintessence Publ. Co.

22. Seymour, R.A., and Walton, J.G. 1984. Pain control after third molar surgery. *Int. J. Oral Surg.* 13:457–485.

23. Curran, J.B., Kennett, S., and Young, A.R. 1974. An assessment of the use of prophylactic antibiotics in third molar surgery. *Int. J. Oral Surg.* 3:1–6.

24. Martis, C., and Karabouta, I. 1984. Infection after orthognathic surgery, with and without preventive antibiotics. *Int. J. Oral Surg.* 13:490–494.

25. Maeglin, B. 1985. Allgemeine chirurgische Grundlagen und Komplikationen bei der Implantation. *Schweiz. Mschr. Zahnmed.* 95:838–840.

26. Interpore International. 1987. *Interpore IMZ Technique Manual.* Revision 3. Irvine, Calif.: Interpore International.

27. Patrick, D., Zosky, J., Lubar, R., and Buchs, A. (In press, 1990.) The longitudinal clinical efficacy of Core-Vent dental implants: A five-year report. *J. Oral Implant.*

28. Calcitek Inc. 1988. Integral biointegrated dental implants. Instructions for use phase 1: implant placement for Integral® (4.0 mm Diameter).

29. Schulte, W. 1981. Das enossale Tübinger Implantat aus Al203 (Frialit®). Der Entwicklungsstand nach 6 Jahren. *Zahnärztl. Mitt.* 71:1181–1192.

30. Maeglin, B. 1988. Allgemeine chirurgische Prinzipien. *In* A. Schroeder, F. Sutter, and G. Krekeler: *Orale Implantologie. Allgemeine Grundlagen und ITI-Hohlzylindersystem.* Stuttgart: Thieme.

31. Burke, J.F. 1973. Preventive antibiotic management in surgery. *Ann. Rev. Med.* 24:289–294.

32. Peterson, L.J. 1984. Antibiotics: Their use in therapy and prophylaxis. *In* G.O. Kruger (ed.) *Oral and Maxillofacial Surgery.* St. Louis: The C.V. Mosby Co.

33. Kaiser, A.B. 1986. Antimicrobial prophylaxis in surgery. *N. Engl. J. Med.* 315:1129–1138.

34. Burke, J.F. 1961. The effective period of preventive antibiotic action in experimental incisions and dermal lesions. *Surgery* 124:268–276.

35. Shulman, S.T., Amren, D.P., Bisno, A.L., et al. 1984. Prevention of bacterial endocarditis. A statement for health professionals by the Committee on Rheumatic Fever and Infective Endocarditis of the Council on Cardiovascular Disease in the Young. American Heart Association Committee of Prevention of Bacterial Endocarditis. *Circulation* 70:1123A–1127A.

36. Nelson, C.L., Green, T.G., Porter, R.A., and Warren, R.D. 1983. One day versus seven days of preventive antibiotic therapy in orthopedic surgery. *Clin. Orthop.* 176:258–263.

37. Conte, J.E., Jr., Cohen, S.N., Roe, B.B., and Elashoff, R.M. 1972. Antibiotic prophylaxis and cardiac surgery: A prospective double-blind comparison of single-dose versus multiple-dose regimen. *Ann. Intern. Med.* 76:943–949.

38. Stone, H.H., Hanney, B.B., Kolb, L.D., Geheber, C.E., and Hooper, C.A. 1979. Prophylactic and

preventive antibiotic therapy: Timing, duration and economics. *Ann. Surg.* 189:691–699.

39. Adell, R., Lekholm, U., Rocker, B., and Brånemark, P.-I. 1981. A 15-year study of osseointegrated implants in the treatment of the edentulous jaw. *Int. J. Oral Surg.* 10:387–416.

40. Kenney, E.B., Weinlander, M., and Moy, P. 1989. Uncovering implants. A review of the UCLA modification of second stage surgical techniques for uncovering implants. *Calif. Dent. Assoc. J.* 17:18–21.

41. Sanz, M., Newman, M.G., Anderson, L., Matoska, W., Otomo-Corgel, J., and Saltini, C. 1989. Clinical enhancement of post periodontal surgical therapy by a 0.12% chlorhexidine gluconate mouthrinse. *J. Periodontol.* 60:570.

42. Newman, M.G., Sanz, M., Nachnani, S., Saltini, C., and Anderson, L. 1989. Effect of 0.12% chlorhexidine on bacterial recolonization following periodontal surgery. *J. Periodontol.* 60:577.

43. Langebaek, J., and Bay, L. 1976. The effect of chlorhexidine mouthrinse on healing after gingivectomy. *Scand. J. Dent. Res.* 84:224–228.

44. Helgeland, K., Heyden, G., and Rölla, G. 1971. Effect of chlorhexidine on animal cells in vitro. *Scand. J. Dent. Res.* 79:209–215.

45. Goldschmidt, P., Cogen, R., and Taubman, S. 1977. Cytopathologic effects of chlorhexidine on human cells. *J. Periodontol.* 48:212–215.

46. Boyed, R.L., Murray, P.A., and Robertson, P.B. 1989. Effect on periodontal status of rotary electric toothbrushes versus manual toothbrushes during periodontal maintenance. I. Clinical results. *J. Periodontol.* 60:390–395.

47. Murray, P.A., Boyed, R.L., and Robertson, P.B. 1989. Effect on periodontal status of rotary electric toothbrushes versus manual toothbrushes during periodontal maintenance. II. Clinical results. *J. Periodontol.* 60:396–401.

48. Flemmig, T.F., Berwick, R.H.F., Newman, M.G., Kenney, E.B., Beumer, J., Nachnani, S. (In press, 1990.) Nep Effekt von Recall auf die subgingivale Mikroflora von osseointegrierten Implantaten. *Z. Zahnärztl. Implant.*

49. Berwick, R.H.F., Flemmig, T.F., Kenney, E.B., Beumer, J., Newman, M.G., Nep, R., Nachnani, S. 1989. Maintenance of gingival health around Brånemark fixtures with UCLA abutment. *J. Dent. Res.* 68:912 (Abstr. no. 365).

50. Schilli, W., and Krekeler, G. 1984. *Der verlagerte Zahn.* Berlin: Quintessenz Verlags.

51. Peterson, L.J. 1987. Principles of antibiotic therapy. *In* R.G. Topazian and M.H. Goldberg (eds.) *Oral and Maxillofacial Infections.* 2nd ed. Philadelphia: W.B. Saunders Co.

52. Lekholm, U., Adell, R., and Brånemark, P.-I. 1985. Possible complications. *In* P-I. Brånemark, G.A. Zarb, and T. Albrektsson (eds.) *Tissue-Integrated Prostheses: Osseointegration in Clinical Dentistry.* Chicago: Quintessence Publ. Co.

53. Adell, R., Lekholm, U., Rockler, B., Brånemark, P.-I., Lindhe, J., Ericsson, B., and Sbordone, L. 1986. Marginal tissue reactions at osseointegrated titanium fixtures. I. A three-year longitudinal prospective study. *Int. J. Oral Surg.* 15:39–52.

54. Lamster, I.B., Alfano, M.C., Seiger, M.C., and Gordon, J.M. 1983. The effect of Listerine Antiseptic® on reduction of existing plaque and gingivitis. *Clin. Prevent. Dent.* 5:12–16.

55. Löe, H., Schiött, C.R., Glavind, L., and Karring, T. 1976. Two years oral use of chlorhexidine in man. I. General design and clinical effects. *J. Periodont. Res.* 17:135–144.

56. Flemmig, T.F., Newman, M.G., Doherty, F.M., Grossman, E., Meckel, A.H., and Bakdash, M.B. 1990. Supragingival irrigation with 0.06% chlorhexidine in naturally occuring gingivitis. I. 6 month clinical observations. *J. Periodontol.* 61:112.

57. Newman, M.G., Flemmig, T.F., Nachnani, S., Rodrigues, A., Calsina, G., Lee, Y-S., de Carmargo, P., Doherty, F.M., and Bakdash, M.B. (In press, 1990.) Supragingival irrigation with 0.06% chlorhexidine in naturally occuring gingivitis. II. 6 months microbiological observations. *J. Periodontol.*

58. Jolkovsky, D.L., Waki, M., Madison, M., Otomo-Corgel, J., Newman, M.G., Nachnani, S., and Flemmig, T.F. 1989. Clinical and microbiological effects of gingival margin irrigation with chlorhexidine. *J. Dent. Res.* 69:970 (Abstr. no. 824).

59. Doherty, F.M., Nachnani, S., Newman, M.G., Hernichel, E., and Sousa, P.R. 1989. Clinical and

microbiological effects of 0.12% chlorhexidine following periodontal maintenance. *J. Dent. Res.* 68:970 (Abstr. no. 825).

60. Krekeler, G., Schilli, W., and Diemer, J. 1985. Should the exit of the artificial abutment tooth be positioned in the region of the attached gingiva? *Int. J. Oral Surg.* 14:504–508.

61. Jovanovic, S.A., Richter, E.-J., and Spiekermann, H. (In press, 1990.) Topographie von periimplantären Knocheneinbrüchen und Theraphieansätze. *Z. Zahnärztl. Implantol.*

62. Dahlin, C., Sennerby, L., Lekholm, U., Lindhe, A., Nyman, S. 1989. Generation of new bone around titanium implants using a membrane technique: An experimental study in rabbits. *Int. J. Oral Maxillofac. Implants* 4:19–25.

63. Duckworth, J., Brose, M., Aver, R., French, C., and Savitt, E. 1987. Therapeutic implications of the bacterial pathogens associated around dental implants. *J. Dent. Res.* 66:144 (Abstr. no. 57).

64. Albrektsson, T. 1988. A multicenter report on osseointegrated oral implants. *J. Prosthet. Dent.* 60:75–84.

PART 5
SPECIAL CONSIDERATIONS

CHAPTER 17

Prophylactic Antibiotic Use

Joan Otomo-Corgel, D.D.S., M.P.H.
Stephen Sonis, D.M.D.

Warning It is not possible to make recommendations regarding antibiotic prophylaxis for all clinical situations. Practitioners should consult with the patient's attending physician(s) before providing dental care. Any unusual clinical event should be noted and corrected immediately.[1]

Antibiotic prophylaxis

Antibiotic prophylaxis is defined as the administration of antibiotics to patients who have no known infection in order to prevent microbial colonization and reduce the potential of postoperative complications. The principles behind the selection of a regimen of antibiotic prophylaxis are listed in **Table 17.1**.

Table 17.1 Principles of antibiotic prophylaxis

- Benefits from prophylaxis outweigh the risks of antibiotic-related allergy, toxicity, superinfection, and development of drug-resistant microbial strains.[2]
- An antibiotic loading dose should be used.
- The antibiotic should be selected as based on the most likely organism to cause an infection.[3]
- Before spread of microorganisms, the antibiotic should be present in blood and target tissues.[4]
- Antibiotic prophylaxis should be continued as long as contamination from the operative site persists.[5]

Bacteremia leading to colonization

Dental causes of bacteremia It is well established that any procedure resulting in gingival bleeding may produce significant bacteremia.[6] Bacteremias have been documented after routine examination procedures, periodontal probing, prophylaxis, and after brushing, flossing, and use of pulsating-pressure irrigating devices. Both the degree of tissue manipulation and the status of oral health influence the magnitude of the bacteremia. Patients with gingival inflammation and periodontal disease develop significantly greater bacteremias, in spectra and amount of bacteria released, than do patients with clean, healthy mouths.

Colonization In the healthy patient, bacteremias appear to be of little clinical importance. However, in the patient who has a condition that predisposes to localized bacterial colonization following bacteremia, a potentially life-threatening situation can develop.[7]

Infective endocarditis

Etiology In infective endocarditis (IE), bacteria, mycoplasmas, fungi, rickettsiae, or chlamydias that are introduced into the blood colonize and multiply on the defective part or roughened surface of the heart. Areas of low blood flow and high turbulence are especially susceptible to bacterial colonization. An endocarditis results, with subsequent stenosis of the mitral valve. The most frequently documented source of bacteremia causing this condition is the oral cavity. Streptococci of the viridans type are most often implicated.

Some studies, however, have detected a decline in streptococcal IE[8,9] and an increase in IE due to *Staphylococcus aureus, Staphylococcus epidermidis,* and HACEK microorganisms (*Hemophilus influenza, Actinobacillus actinomycetemcomitans, Cardiobacterium hominis, Eikenella corrodens, Kingella kingii*).[8]

Susceptible patients Experts on the subject of IE and patient susceptibility have not reached uniform consensus on risk categorization. Pallasch[10] has developed an at-risk table with categories based on potential for bacteremia and risk:benefit ratios for antibiotic efficacy versus toxicity (see **Table 17.2**). The American Heart Association recommends prophylactic antibiotic coverage with the **Special Regimen** for four categories of very-high-risk patients: *(1)* previous history of IE, *(2)* cardiac valve prosthesis, *(3)* coarctation of the aorta, and *(4)* indwelling catheter left side of the heart.

Premedication

Penicillin Fortunately, the majority of organisms that cause IE are generally suscepti-

---

Table 17.2   Patients at-risk from bacteremia-induced infections*

Very-high-risk, high-risk, and intermediate-risk patients should receive antibiotic prophylaxis. No chemoprophylaxis is normally required for low-risk patients.† Other indications may include orthopedic prosthetic appliances, hemodialysis, and impaired host defenses.

Antibiotic prophylaxis indicated

Very high risk

Previous episode of infective endocarditis
Heart valve prosthesis
Coarctation of the aorta
Indwelling catheter left side of heart

High risk

Rheumatic heart disease
Other acquired valvular heart disease
Congenital heart disease
   Ventricular septal defect
   Patent ductus arteriosus
   Tetralogy of Failot
   Complex cyanotic heart disease
   Systemic-pulmonary artery shunt
   Indwelling catheter right side of heart
   Mitral valve surgery
   Mitral valve prolapse with murmur
   Ventriculoatrial shunts for hydrocephalus
   Idiopathic hypertrophic subaortic stenosis

Intermediate risk

Tricuspid valve disease
Assymetric septal hypertrophy

Other at-risk patients

Orthopedic prosthetic devices
Immunosuppression
Hemodialysis

Antibiotic prophylaxis usually not indicated†

Low risk

Mitral valve prolapse without murmur
Coronary artery disease
Atherosclerotic plaque
Previous myocardial infarction

Coronary bypass

Indwelling cardiac pacemakers
Congenital pulmonary stenosis
Uncomplicated secundum septal atrial defect
Six months or longer after surgery for:
   Ligated ductus arteriosus
   Autogenous vascular grafts
   Surgically closed atrial or septal defects
      (without Dacron patches)

---

*Reprinted with permission of Pallasch. [10]
†Check with patient's physician.

ble to penicillin, although some notable exceptions occur. The current recommendations by the American Heart Association were formulated some years ago (1984) and are penicillin-based (see **Table 17.3**).[11] Recently, the Advisory Board of the Medical Letter, an authoritative and timely publication, changed their recommendation to an amoxicillin-based regimen based on the favorable uptake and spectrum properties of the drug. Amoxicillin has been successfully used for IE prophylaxis for some time in the United Kingdom.

   The AHA has established two regimens for IE prophylaxis based on the patient's expected risk for IE. The oral regimen is applicable for patients at low or moderate risk

Table 17.3 Recommended antibiotic regimens for prevention of infective endocarditis during dental and upper respiratory procedures

Adult dosage	Children's dosage
Standard regimen	**Standard regimen**
2 g of penicillin V 1 h preoperatively; 1 g, 6 h after the initial dose.	>60 lb—adult dosage <60 lb—one half the adult dose 1 h before the procedure and 6 h after the initial dose
Penicillin-allergic	Penicillin-allergic
1.6 g of erythromycin ethylsuccinate 1.5 h preoperatively; 0.8 g, 6 h after the initial dose.	20 mg/kg of erythromycin ethylsuccinate 1.5 h before the procedure and 6 h after the initial dose
(If base or sterate forms of erythromycin are used, adequate blood levels will probably not be reached in the initial 1 h preoperative recommendation.) 1 g erythromycin 1 h preoperatively; 500 mg 6 h after the initial dose.	
Special regimen	**Special regimen**
Ampicillin 1–2 g IM or IV plus gentamicin 1.5 mg/kg IM or IV 30–60 min preoperatively. 1 g of penicillin V 6 h after the initial dose or repeat the parenteral regimen 8 h later.	Ampicillin 50 mg/kg IM or IV 30–60 min before procedure then repeat once 8 h later. Gentamicin 20 mg/kg IM or IV 30–60 min before procedure then repeat once 8 h later either parenterally or orally (1 g of penicillin V).
Penicillin-allergic	Penicillin-allergic
Vancomycin 1 g IV administered slowly over 1 h starting 1 h before treatment; no postoperative dose required.	Vancomycin 20 mg/kg IV infused over 1 h, beginning 1 h before procedure.

and consists of penicillin VK 2 g per os 1 hour preoperatively followed by a second dose of 1 g 6 hours later. Alternatively, the Medical Letter suggests amoxicillin 3 g 1 hour preoperatively followed by 1.5 g 6 hours later. Erythromycin, 1 g 1½ to 2 hours preoperatively, followed by 500 mg 6 hours after the initial dose can be used in patients allergic to penicillin or by patients taking daily penicillin for streptococcal prophylaxis following rheumatic fever.

For patients at high risk of IE (see **Table 17.4**), initial parenteral antibiotic therapy is indicated.

While the AHA regimens call for a single postoperative dose of antibiotic, continuation of antibiotic therapy should be considered in any procedure following which a prolonged bacteremia is likely. Among these are extractions, biopsies,

Table 17.4 Relative risks of infective endocarditis based on underlying cardiac lesions and American Heart Association recommended protocol

At-risk level	Recommended protocol
Patients at high risk:	Special regimen (see **Table 17.3**)
• Previous history of IE • Prosthetic heart valve • Intravascular prostheses • Coarctation of the aorta	
Patients at significant risk:	Standard regimen (see **Table 17.3**)
• Rheumatic valvular diseases • Acquired valvular disease • Congenital heart disease	
Patients at minimal risk:	Standard regimen (see **Table 17.3**)
• Transvenous pacemaker • History of rheumatic fever without rheumatic heart disease	
Patients with minimal risk who do not usually require prophylaxis:*	Standard regimen (see **Table 17.3**)
• Incurred or functional murmur • Uncomplicated atical septal defects • Coronary artery bypass graft operations	

*Check with patient's physician.

periodontal surgery and endodontic therapy in an infected area. For patients requiring suture removal, which is likely to produce bleeding, it is prudent to continue patients on a therapeutic level of antibiotic postoperatively, rather than to start and stop and start on prophylaxis dose of antibiotic over a short period or to use resorbable sutures.

Penicillin-allergic patients Erythromycin is the oral antibiotic of choice for patients allergic to penicillin. **Vancomycin** can be used for parenteral administration in penicillin-allergic individuals.

Patients with special considerations

Two groups of patients who require alteration of antibiotic prophylaxis for IE are: *(1)* patients who take daily penicillin as prophylaxis and *(2)* patients with localized juvenile periodontitis (LJP) who are susceptible.

In the past, patients taking penicillin daily have been treated preoperatively with additional doses of penicillin. However, recent data suggest that penicillin-resistant organisms may develop and that prophylaxis with erythromycin should be considered in this group.[12] The same daily dose as for penicillin should be maintained.

Patients with LJP have been shown to have increased numbers of penicillin-resistant *Actinobacillus actinomycetemcomitans,* known to produce infective endocarditis, present in periodontal lesions. Pretreatment with 250 mg of tetracycline four times a day for 2 weeks, followed by the regular recommended prophylaxis medication, has been recommended. Tetracycline is very effective against *Actinobacillus.*[13] Consult with the patient's physician. An alternative regimen of metronidazole plus Augmentin (250 mg tid of each) for 3 days is effective against *A. actinomycetemcomitans.*[14]

When to premedicate

Any potential cardiac problem suspected in a patient warrants consultation with the patient's physician *before* beginning treatment. **If in doubt, premedicate**. The worst possible outcome is allergy and/or resistance. Although the incidence of IE is low (approximately 1% of all cardiac disorders), it is a serious disease with a poor prognosis despite modern therapy.

Renal disease

Renal transplant recipients and hemodialysis patients need prophylactic antibiotic therapy before dental treatment.[15] Consultation with the patient's physician is prudent to determine the patient's renal function, degree of immunosuppression, presence of concomitant disease, and to discuss antibiotic choice. In general, penicillin or erythromycin may be used for prophylaxis in this group of patients.

Hemodialysis

Hemodialysis removes impurities from the blood of patients with chronic renal failure. Blood is channeled from an artery to a dialysis machine, where it is cleaned and then sent back to the veins. An arteriovenous shunt is surgically created to accomplish this. Premedication is needed before dental procedures because the shunt is susceptible to bacterial implantation and infection following bacteremia. The regimen recommended for IE prophylaxis is usually acceptable for these patients.

Renal transplant

With the exception of grafts between siblings, renal transplants are allografts. Although there may be differences in compatibility depending on the donor source, immunosuppression of recipients is always required to maximize the chances of graft survival. *Thus, renal transplant recipients receive chronic doses of corticosteroids, usually prednisone, and may receive short courses of cytotoxic drugs such as cytoxan during rejection episodes. As a consequence of chronic immunosuppression, transplant recipients are susceptible to infection and therefore require antibiotic prophylaxis before dental treatment and aggressive treatment of dental infection.*

The course of antibiotics recommended for IE prophylaxis may be adequate for most patients; however, some physicians prefer more aggressive antibiotic prophylaxis, especially when surgical procedures are contemplated, as in patients at risk for IE prophylaxis, where antibiotic coverage should be continued during the postoperative period during which healing occurs. **It is crucial that the dentist and physician communicate before dental treatment.**

Joint prosthesis

An association has been suggested between dental manipulation and late, nonoperation-associated infection of joint prostheses used in total hip replacement.[16] It is speculated that the bacteremia resulting from dental treatment seeds the prosthesis and produces infection. However, the evidence is circumstantial at best and the association may only be coincidental. No guidelines have been developed relating to antibiotic premedication of the prosthetic joint.[17,18] However, until a definitive examination of the subject has been completed, it is prudent for these patients to receive antibiotic prophylaxis before dental treatment. The consequences of infection of the prosthesis far outweigh the risk of antibiotic sensitivity.

Premedication for joint prostheses   What *form* antibiotic prophylaxis should take is controversial. For many years, the standard prophylaxis used for the prevention of IE was recommended. However, a recent study that determined the identity and drug sensitivity of the causative organisms demonstrated that *S. aureus* **is the most common offending organism to patients with artificial joints.**[19]

It appears prudent that the prophylactic regimen should include an antistaphylococcal agent (cephalosporin or antistaphylococcal penicillin). However, because streptococci are the bacteria cultured during transient bacteremia from a dental/oral manipulation, should penicillin be the preferred drug? The controversy is evident among orthopedic surgeons an well. For example, a survey among orthopedic surgeons indicated that 57.3% of respondents felt dental-induced bacteremia and orthopedic hip infections were minimal or not important. Paradoxically, 93% indicated they recommended antibiotic prophylaxis before dental treatments.[18]

Because many of these organisms are penicillin-resistant, the authors suggest that erythromycin, clindamycin, or a β-lactamase-resistant penicillin be used for prophylaxis. **Consult with the patient's orthopedic surgeon before performing any dental procedure that may cause bleeding (many surgeons tend to prefer cephalosporins).**

Other diseases

Diminished capacity to fight infection   Patients with a variety of other systemic disorders, as well as the very young or very old, may have a diminished capacity to deal with infection. Antibiotic prophylaxis before dental manipulation may be desirable for **patients with diabetes mellitus, cancer, Down's syndrome, or cirrhosis of the liver; patients receiving steroids; splenectomized individuals[20]; and patients with impaired host defenses.** Patients with acquired immunodeficiency virus should not receive antibiotic prophylaxis due to potential development of antibiotic-resistant organisms that could create serious infection.

In each of these cases, communication with the patient's physician is imperative to determine the status of the patient's systemic disease and to assess his or her ability to deal with potentially infectious organisms.

Determining need   The need for prophylaxis may depend on the extent of the anticipated procedure. Antibiotic prophylaxis similar to that used for cardiac disease patients is recommended in any case where there is doubt, because infection in compromised patients can have serious consequences. Early identification of the offending organism(s) followed by aggressive, specific antibiotic therapy, is recommended. Prophylactic antibiotics to reduce postoperative infection from dental procedures is probably of little or no value.

Conclusion

Further research and evaluation of the use of antibiotics for the purpose of prophylaxis before dental procedures is greatly needed. When there is minimal inflammation there is minimal to nondiscernible bacteremia. Preoperative de-germing (e.g., with chlorhexidine gluconate) may reduce bacteremia.[21] A high level of oral hygiene reduces bacteremia, yet oral hygiene instrumentation may induce bacteremia. The dental professional should recognize the implications and indications of antibiotic prophylaxis. Attempts should be made to continually reduce inflammation in oral tissues and to minimize antibiotics during dental therapy.

References

1. Ciancio, S.G. 1980. *Clinical Pharmacology for Dental Professionals.* New York: McGraw-Hill Book Co., p. 289.
2. Polk, H.C., Jr., and Lopez-Mayor, J.R. 1969. Postoperative wound infection: A prospective study of

determinant factors and prevention. *Surgery* 66:97.

3. Weinstein, L. 1954. The chemoprophylaxis of infection. *Ann. Intern. Med.* 43:287.

4. *The Medical Letter on Drugs and Therapeutics.* Antibiotic prophylaxis for surgery. 1985. 27:105.

5. Burke, J.F. 1961. The effective period of preventive antibiotic action in experimental incisions and dermal lesions. *Surgery* 50:61.

6. Crawford, J.J., et al. 1974. Bacteremia after tooth extraction studied with the aid of prereduced anaerobically sterilized culture media. *Appl. Microbiol.* 27:927–932.

7. Sipes, J.N., Thompson, R.I., and Hook, E.W. 1977. Prophylaxis of infective endocarditis: A reevaluation. *Am. Rev. Med.* 38:371.

8. Brandenburg, R.O., Giuliani, E.R., Wilson, W.R., et al. 1983. Infective endocarditis—A 25 year overview of diagnosis and therapy. *J. Am. Coll. Cardiol.* 1:280.

9. Gossius, G., Gunnes, P., and Rasmussen, K. 1985. Ten years of infective endocarditis: A clinico-pathologic study. *Acta Med. Scand.* 217:171.

10. Pallasch, T.J. 1989. Antibiotic prophylaxis: Theory and reality. *CDA Journal* 17:27–39.

11. Committee on Rheumatic Fever and Infective Endocarditis of the Council on Cardiovascular Disease in the Young. 1984. Prevention of bacterial endocarditis: A statement for health professionals. *Circulation* 70:1123A–1127A.

12. Parillo, J.E., et al. 1979. Endocarditis due to resistant Viridans streptococci during penicillin prophylaxis. *New Engl. J. Med.* 300:296.

13. Slots, J., Bengt, R.G., and Genco, R. 1983. Suppression of penicillin resistant oral *Actinobacillus actinomycetemcomitans* with tetracycline: Considerations in endocarditis prophylaxis. *J. Periodontol.* 54:193–196.

14. van Winkelhoff, A.J., Rodenburg, J.P., et al. 1989. Metronidazole plus amoxicillin in the treatment of *Actinobacillus actinomycetemcomitans* associated periodontitis. *J. Clin. Periodontol.* 16:128–131.

15. Tyldesley, W.R., Rotter, E., and Sells, R.A. 1979. Oral lesions in renal transplant patients. *J. Oral Pathol.* 8:53.

16. Rubin, R., Salvati, E.A., and Lewis, R., 1976. Infected total hip replacement after dental procedures. *Oral Surg.* 41:18.

17. Little, J.W. 1983. The need for antibiotic coverage for dental treatment of patients with joint replacements. *Oral Surg. Oral Med. Oral Pathol.* 55:20.

18. Jaspers, M.T., and Little, J. 1985. Prophylaxis antibiotic coverage in patients with total arthroplasty: Current practice. *J. Am. Dent. Assoc.* 111:943–948.

19. Jacobsen, P.L., and Murray, W. 1980. Prophylactic coverage of dental patients with artificial joints: A retrospective analysis of thirty-three infections in hip prostheses. *Oral Surg.* 50:49.

20. Quintiliani, R., and Maderazo, E.G. 1981. Infections in the compromised patient. *In* R.G. Topazian and M.G. Goldberg (eds.) *Management of Infections of the Oral and Maxillofacial Regions.* Philadelphia: W.B. Saunders Co.

21. Bender, I.B., and Barkan, M.J. 1989. Dental bacteremia and its relationship to endocarditis: Preventive measures. *Contin. Educ. Dent.* 10:472–482.

CHAPTER 18

Antimicrobial Therapy for Immunocompromised Patients

Spencer W. Redding, D.D.S., M.Ed.

Patients who suffer from immunosuppression commonly develop serious oral infections of both hard and soft tissues. This chapter will focus on three groups of immunocompromised patients: *(1)* those receiving cancer chemotherapy, *(2)* those with HIV infection, and *(3)* those receiving organ transplantation. Cancer chemotherapy will be discussed first and used as a model for the development of oral infection. Then HIV infection and organ transplantation will be compared to cancer chemotherapy.

Cancer chemotherapy

Cancer chemotherapy is a commonly used modality to treat certain types of cancer primarily and other types of cancer adjunctively. The destruction of rapidly dividing cancer cells is the goal of cancer chemotherapy. Cells undergoing growth and division are more sensitive to the effects of chemotherapy than are resting cells. Normal cells that rapidly divide are susceptible to the effects of chemotherapy and can be destroyed. These cells include bone marrow, gastrointestinal mucosa, reproductive cells, and hair. The effects of chemotherapy lead to a reduction of protective cells produced by the bone marrow, resulting in the complications of oral infection. These infections can be divided into odontogenic infections and soft tissue infections.[1]

Odontogenic infection (see Table 18.1)

Odontogenic infection, including periapical, periodontal, and pericoronal infections, can lead to significant morbidity in the patient on cancer chemotherapy. Neutropenia (less than 2,000 circulating neutrophils) is a common complication of chemotherapy and has been shown to predispose those patients to systemic infection. Therefore, an odontogenic infection that would be limited to the oral cavity in an otherwise healthy patient can undergo systemic spread in the patient on cancer chemotherapy. It has been

---

Table 18.1   Principles for managing odontogenic infections in patients undergoing cancer chemotherapy

---

- Eliminate all potential sources of odontogenic infection before chemotherapy
- Use prophylactic antibiotics (see **Table 18.2**) for all dental procedures:
  (1) in patients with a neutrophil count less than 2,000 or
  (2) in patients who have received chemotherapy within the previous 2 wk
- Prophylactic antibiotics should be given *before* dental therapy and 6 h postoperatively
- Prophylaxis should be extended for at least 5 d postoperatively if a major surgical procedure is performed

---

shown that odontogenic infection can be a significant source of septicemia in this patient population.[2] Because of this potential for spread of infection, it is imperative that patients have all potential sources of odontogenic infection eliminated before starting cancer chemotherapy.

Because these patients will become neutropenic within 7 to 10 days after the initiation of their chemotherapy, the use of prophylactic antibiotics with dental manipulation must be considered. This antibiotic coverage must be discussed with the patient's oncologist. All patients with a neutrophil count of less than 2,000 or who will shortly develop neutropenia should be considered for prophylaxis. With cancer chemotherapy there is commonly a shift toward more gram-negative bacteria in the oral cavity. Therefore it is important to include antibiotic coverage for these organisms. Traditionally this has included the use of a synthetic penicillin such as **ticarcillin** and an aminoglycoside such as gentamicin. The antibiotics should be given just before dental therapy to achieve an adequate blood level and should be given postoperatively, preferably 6 hours after treatment. If active infection is present or if a major surgical procedure is involved, extension of this prophylaxis to a period of 5 days should be considered (see **Table 18.2**).

Mucositis

Patients receiving cancer chemotherapy commonly develop mucositis of the soft tissues of the oral cavity. This mucositis is secondary to the toxic effects of chemotherapy on the oral epithelium, but the mucositis can be complicated or secondarily infected with bacteria, candidal organisms, and herpes simplex virus. Candidal infections can be diagnosed by the use of Gram's staining or potassium hydroxide staining. If these are found to be positive, the patient should be treated with **nystatin, clotrimazole,** or **ketoconazole** (refer to **Table 18.2** for correct therapy; see also chapters 5 and 8).

Patients with mucositis should also be evaluated for the presence of herpes simplex virus. In immunocompromised patients, such as those on cancer chemotherapy, a very high percentage of patients (as high as 50% of those being treated for leukemia) will

Table 18.2   Antimicrobial therapy with cancer chemotherapy

Infection/virus	Treatment
Odontogenic	If neutropenic, treat with ticarcillin 3 g plus gentamicin 1.5 mg/kg IV before therapy and then repeat dosage 6 h later (treat for longer duration if active infection or if major surgical procedure is involved)
Candidiasis	*Nystatin suspension:* swish in mouth for 2 min and swallow 4 times/d for 14 d
	Clotrimazole troches: dissolve 1 troche in mouth 5 times/d for 14 d
	Ketoconazole: take 1 tablet daily for 14 d
Herpes simplex	*Acyclovir IV:* 5 mg/kg given over 1 h 3 times/d for 5–7 d
	Acyclovir capsules: take 1 capsule 5 times/d for 7–10 d
	Acyclovir prophylaxis for bone marrow transplant: take acyclovir capsules 3 times/d the day before transplant, continue for 6 wk; if patient develops severe oral mucositis, switch to IV form 5 mg/kg 3 times/d; when mucositis resolves, switch back to capsules
Mucositis	*0.12% chlorhexidine rinse:* 7 mL for 30 s 3 times/d beginning the day before therapy and continuing until mucositis resolves

reactivate herpes simplex virus in the presence of their oral mucositis. These lesions are very severe and can involve any soft tissue surface in and around the oral cavity.[3] The mucositis lesions should be evaluated for herpes simplex virus, preferably by culturing. When found to be positive, these patients should be treated with **acyclovir** (refer to **Table 18.2** for recommended therapy; see also chapters 5 and 8). Inpatients with severe disease should be initially treated with the intravenous form of acyclovir; those to be maintained as outpatients with less severe disease should be treated with acyclovir capsules.[4]

Bone marrow transplantation

A subset of patients receiving high-dose cancer chemotherapy are those undergoing bone marrow transplantation. These patients receive very high doses of chemotherapy, which destroy the bone marrow. Therefore, these patients will suffer the same complications as patients receiving conventional chemotherapy but the complications are often much more severe. All the above evaluations apply to these patients. Because of the incidence of reactivation of herpes simplex virus (in some studies over 80%), **acyclovir** prophylaxis is commonly used. Patients are evaluated before transplant, and if found to have positive antibodies to herpes simplex virus, they receive acyclovir prophylaxis through their therapy (refer to **Table 18.2** for treatment recommendations).

The use of antimicrobial mouthrinse therapy may have an indication in patients on high-dose cancer chemotherapy. It has been shown that prophylactic rinsing with chlorhexidine in bone marrow transplant patients can reduce the severity of oral mucositis and also reduce the incidence of candidal infections[5] (refer to **Table 18.2** for appropriate therapy for use of chlorhexidine).

HIV infection

Patients infected with the human immunodeficiency virus (HIV) very commonly present with oral opportunistic infections. Several of these infections, such as candidiasis and herpes simplex reactivation, are early diagnostic predictors of disease progression.

Odontogenic infection

Odontogenic infection can be a significant problem in these patients. Periapical and pericoronal infection should be treated very aggressively either by root canal therapy or extraction. The patient who develops these infections and is HIV positive but whose immune system appears to be adequate can be treated as a normal dental patient. However, when a patient has developed the immune system changes secondary to HIV infection (i.e., AIDS has been diagnosed), antibiotic coverage should be strongly considered as an adjunct in the treatment of odontogenic infections. Oral penicillin should be the drug of choice and should be given before therapy and at least 6 hours after. If active infection is present, an increase in the duration of the penicillin to 5 days should be considered (see **Table 18.2**).

HIV-gingivitis/HIV-periodontitis

Patients with HIV infection have been found to develop a distinctive type of gingivitis and periodontal disease. These are currently termed HIV-gingivitis and HIV-periodontitis. It appears critical that HIV-gingivitis be treated aggressively at this stage because once the patient develops HIV-periodontitis it is very difficult to treat. It has also been shown that the aggressive therapy of HIV-gingivitis can prevent periodontitis from occurring. Aggressive scaling and root planing combined with **chlorhexidine** rinsing has been found to be an effective therapy in both gingivitis and periodontitis patients (see **Table 18.3** for appropriate therapy). Periodontitis patients who do not respond to this initial therapy may receive a benefit from a course of oral **metronidazole**.[6,7]

Oral candidiasis

Virtually all HIV patients will develop oral candidiasis at some time during their

---

Table 18.3 Antimicrobial therapy with HIV infection and organ transplantation

---

Infection/virus	Treatment
Odontogenic	Penicillin VK 2 g orally 1 h before treatment and then 1 g 6 h later (treat for longer duration if active infection or major surgical procedure involved)
HIV gingivitis/ periodontitis	Vigorous scaling and root planing and 0.12% chlorhexidine rinse 7 mL for 30 s 3 times/d for 7 d
	If above is unsuccessful, metronidazole 250-mg tablets 4 times/d for 7 d
Candidiasis	*Nystatin suspension:* swish in mouth for 2 min and swallow 4 times/d for 14 d
	Clotrimazole troches: dissolve 1 troche in mouth 5 times/d for 14 d
	Ketoconazole: take 1 tablet daily for 14 d
Herpes simplex	*Acyclovir IV:* 5 mg/kg given over 1 h 3 times/d for 5–7 d
	Acyclovir capsules: take 1 capsule 5 times/d for 7–20 d
	Acyclovir prophylaxis for organ transplantation: acyclovir capsules 3 times/d beginning the day of transplant and continue for 30 d

---

disease. This should be diagnosed and treated as discussed above under cancer chemotherapy.

Herpes simplex virus

As many as 25% of HIV positive patients will reactivate herpes simplex virus in and around the oral cavity at some time during their disease. As with cancer chemotherapy, these lesions are atypical, very aggressive, and very painful. These lesions should be treated with intravenous **acyclovir** in the inpatient with severe disease and with acyclovir capsules in the outpatient with less severe disease. Some patients who experience numerous reactivations of herpes simplex virus may be maintained on acyclovir prophylaxis with the oral capsules.

Organ transplantation

Patients who receive organ transplantation must receive immunosuppressive therapy for the rest of their lives to prevent rejection of their new organ. Because of chronic immunosuppression, patients receiving dental care or experiencing odontogenic infection should be prophylaxed with penicillin before and after their therapy. Oral **penicillin** is the drug of choice and should be given as above under HIV infection. These patients will also develop oral candidiasis because of immunosuppression. They should be evaluated and treated as above. Anywhere from 25% to 70% of these patients will reactivate herpes simplex virus in and about the mouth. Commonly, if these patients have positive herpes simplex virus antibody titers before transplant they are placed on acyclovir prophylaxis with their transplant therapy (see **Table 18.3**).

References

1. Peterson, D.E., Elias, E.G., and Sonis, S.T. 1986. *Head and Neck Management of the Cancer Patient.* Boston: Martinus Nijhoff.

2. Greenberg, M.S., et al. 1982. The oral flora as a source of septicemia in patients with acute leukemia. *Oral Surg. Oral Med. Oral Pathol.* 53:32–36.

3. Montgomery, M.T., Redding, S.W., and Le Maistre, C.F. 1986. The incidence of oral herpes simplex virus infection in patients undergoing cancer chemotherapy. *Oral Surg. Oral Med. Oral Pathol.* 61:238–242.

4. Gold, D., and Corey, L. 1987. Acyclovir prophylaxis for herpes simplex virus infection. *Antimicrob. Agents Chemother.* 31:361–367.

5. Feretti, G.A., et al. 1987. Chlorhexidine for prophylaxis against oral infections and associated complications in patients receiving bone marrow transplants. *J. Am. Dent. Assoc.* 114:461–467.

6. Robertson, P.B., and Greenspan, J.S. 1988. *Perspectives on Oral Manifestations of AIDS.* Littleton, Mass.: PSG Publishing Co.

7. Grassi, M., et al. 1988. Local treatments of HIV associated periodontal disease. *J. Dent. Res.* 67:127.

CHAPTER 19

Systemic Considerations for Female Patients

Joan Otomo-Corgel, D.D.S., M.P.H.

Approximately 10 million women are taking oral contraceptives and 60% to 75% of pregnant women will have mild to severe gingivitis. Oral changes may occur during menstruation and before, during, and after menopause. For these women, the occurrence of problematic oral symptoms increases. Therefore, the effects of systemic antimicrobials/antibiotics need particular attention with respect to the female patient's individual ovarian hormone production (estrogen and progesterone). Continual updating of medical histories is a prerequisite because of the diverse systemic reactions to these fluctuating hormonal levels.

Considerations of antibiotic prescription

Vaginitis

A common side effect of antibiotic use is vaginitis. When the vaginal mixed flora is depressed by the presence of an antibiotic, an overgrowth of *Candida* sp. can be produced. A post-menopausal patient is less likely to develop *Candida* infections because the vaginal flora has already been altered by an absence of estrogen.[1] Other bacterial vaginal infections can occur in these patients, however. The older patient's symptoms could be caused by atrophic changes in the vagina that require estrogen therapy as well as antibiotic treatment. If yeast infection/vaginitis occurs, it is best to refer a patient to her gynecologist rather than to risk inappropriate treatment. Many women are aware of the likelihood of vaginitis when they are placed on antibiotics. Consult with the patient's gynecologist as to the feasibility of prophylactic vaginal suppositories (i.e., nystatin) if the antibiotic is necessary for the proposed dental therapy.

Contraceptive failure

Antibiotic use in women has recently been associated with the failure of oral contraceptives (i.e., tetracyclines).[2] The effect of antibiotics on the enterohepatic circulation of contraceptive steroids is proven in animals, but only **rifampin,** an anti-tuberculosis agent, has been shown to cause contraceptive failure in humans by this mechanism.[3,4] An additional mode of action has been proposed. Until further research clarifies this issue, **it is prudent to advise patients using birth control pills that contraceptive failure may occur.**

The pregnant or nursing patient

Selection of an antibiotic for pregnant or nursing women must be made with equal consideration for mother and child. **Antibiotics with systemic effects cross the placenta and reach the fetus.** Drug concentrations in breast milk are usually low, but a neonate's ability to metabolize drugs is undeveloped, especially if he or she was born prematurely.[5-13] Note that the effect of a particular medication on the fetus depends on the type of antimicrobial, dosage, trimester, and duration of the course of therapy.

Table 19.1 summarizes the risks of antibiotic use in pregnant and nursing women.

Antibiotics and their effects in pregnant and lactating women

Penicillin   Penicillin can be used in pregnancy without any known teratogenic effects. Some controversy exists over whether breast-feeding causes sensitization of infants to penicillin. Parents should inform their pediatricians if their children have been nursed by mothers taking penicillin. Ampicillin is excreted in breast milk, though not in therapeutic doses. If an infant develops moniliasis or diarrhea, however, the possible role of ampicillin should be taken into consideration.[5-13]

Aminoglycosides   Aminoglycosides frequently are used for urinary infections during pregnancy and are associated with ototoxicity and nephrotoxicity in the mother. When aminoglycosides have been used in the last trimester, the child should have his or her hearing evaluated. **Aminoglycosides will enter breast milk and, although not absorbed by the infant's gut, may disturb intestinal flora.**[6,12]

Sulfonamides   Sulfonamides are safe to administer in the first and second trimesters of pregnancy, but use during the third trimester or the postpartum period if breast-feeding can lead to **kernicterus** in premature infants. Glucose-6-phosphate dehydrogenase deficiency can result in hemolysis in infants who receive sulfonamides or nitrofurantoins. A family history of G-6-PD deficiency would contraindicate use of sulfonamides and trimethoprim sulfonamide combinations.[5-13]

Erythromycin   Erythromycin is often given to penicillin-sensitive patients. However,

Table 19.1 Risks of antibiotic use in pregnant and lactating women

Drug group	Crosses placenta or enters breast milk	Safe for pregnant or lactating women	Risks
Penicillin	Yes	Yes	Diarrhea in infant, sensitization in infant
Cephalosporin	Yes	Yes (relatively limited information)	Diarrhea in infant
Sulfonamides	Yes	No	Kernicterus in infant, risk with G-6-PD deficiency
Aminoglycosides	Yes	Yes—with caution	Diarrhea in infant and possible ototoxicity
Tetracycline	Yes	No	Affects bone and teeth
Clindamycin	Yes	Yes—with caution	Drug concentrated in fetal bone, spleen, lung, and liver
Chloramphenicol	Yes	No	"Gray syndrome" associated with death in infant at term
Erythromycin	Yes	No	Intrahepatic jaundice in mother
Metronidazole	Yes	No	Theoretical carcinogenic data in animals
Vancomycin	Yes	No	Limited information
Streptomycin	Yes	No	Congenital deafness

erythromycin estolates can cause intrahepatic cholestatic jaundice in the mother and is **contraindicated in pregnancy and lactation.**[5]

Tetracycline **Tetracycline should not be prescribed to pregnant or lactating women.** It accumulates in bones and chelates calcium, inhibiting bone growth and discoloring teeth in the fetus, especially when taken in the last half of pregnancy. Severe hepatotoxicity might also occur in the mother. Infants exposed to tetracycline in breast milk have not shown bone and teeth changes, probably because the tetracycline was chelated by calcium in the breast milk. It is nevertheless contraindicated in lactating women because of the high concentration of the drug in breast milk.[8]

Cephalosporins Cephalosporins will cross the placenta but are not associated with teratogenic effects or with concentrations of the drug in the fetus. Cephalexin (Keflex®) is not believed to be excreted in breast milk in significant amounts.[6,13]

Clindamycin Clindamycin will cross the placenta and appear in the breast milk. It concentrates in fetal liver, kidney, bone, spleen, and lung tissues. Although no bone growth changes have been reported from the drug concentrating, newborns should be examined closely if they were exposed in utero.

Chloramphenicol   Chloramphenicol will cross the placenta and be excreted in breast milk in significant amounts. It cannot be metabolized by an infant's liver and kidney, and if used near term can cause **"gray syndrome,"** which has a high death rate. Chloramphenicol should not be given to nursing mothers because of the underdeveloped enzyme systems of infants. A G-6-PD-deficient infant could contract **neonatal hemolysis** if his or her nursing mother uses chloramphenicol.[5,8]

Metronidazole   Metronidazole crosses the placenta and reaches high concentrations in breast milk. Although there has been no documented fetal damage from its use, data from animal studies have suggested that metronidazole could be carcinogenic.[11] Consult the patient's physician when this agent is considered because of severe or refractory oral infection.

Periodontal considerations

An increase in gingival inflammation and gingival exudate is a common oral manifestation of increased levels of ovarian hormones (estrogen and progesterone).[14] Pregnancy, oral contraceptives, menstruation, and puberty have been documented in relation to transient periods of gingivitis. There is a significant increase in gingivitis and proportions of *Bacteroides melaninogenicus, ss intermedius,** and *ss melaninogenicus** in plaque as pregnancy progresses, with a return to pre-pregnancy levels as sex hormones decline with parturition.[15,16] Studies have demonstrated that estrogens and progesterones applied topically give rise to impaired vascular function,[17] increased vascular permeability,[18] and stimulated vascular proliferation. Progesterone alters microvascular permeability[19] and alters the rate of collagen production (wound healing).[20] Therefore, the increase in hormone levels may predispose the female patient to exaggerated gingival inflammation by enhancing bacterial growth, depression of immune response,[21] and alteration of folate metabolism.[22]

Most clinicians and researchers agree that if the pregnant woman institutes excellent home care and is plaque free at onset of pregnancy, the incidence of gingivitis is low.[23] Antibiotics are not the treatment of choice at initial notice of gingival inflammation. Meticulous removal of irritants and good oral hygiene will eliminate the need for systemic medications. Chlorhexidine gluconate rinsing has not yet been approved for use in the pregnant woman. Note that a female taking oral contraceptives for longer periods of time may develop a chronic gingival inflammation that can predispose her to periodontitis. Close periodontal monitoring should be performed, as should supportive periodontal therapy, maintenance, and home care reinforcement.

If the clinician feels that the need for an antibiotic outweighs the risks, the second trimester and first half of the third trimester are the safest times to treat the pregnant patient.[24] Expanding infection with systemic involvement may require the need for systemic antibiotics.

* Nomenclature used in original article.[15]

Special note: pain medication associated with oral infection

It is frequently asked whether oral pain medications should be given to pregnant and lactating women undergoing painful dental treatment. Postoperative dental pain can be severe and it would be unfair to deprive these patients of pain relief in this acute setting. **Local anesthetics can be used with no ill effects to a fetus.** Some oral medications can also be used to relieve pain. Codeine, although it will cross the placenta and occur in small amounts in breast milk, can be given in therapeutic dosages when required. Acetaminophen can safely be used as a nonnarcotic pain medication, but **aspirin should be avoided during pregnancy and lactation** due to its possible effects on an infant's platelets.[12]

Summary: benefits outweigh risks

It is not logical to ignore or delay treatment of a dental infection during pregnancy because systemic effects of infection could be harmful to mother and fetus. When antibiotics are given during pregnancy or breast-feeding, it is best to coordinate care with an obstetrician or pediatrician. Dangers of bacteremia or septicemia are greater to the fetus than are the dangers that the antibiotic will cross the placenta.

References

1. Friedrich, E. 1976. *Vulvar Disease*. Philadelphia: W.B. Saunders Co., pp. 17–25.
2. Back, D.J., et al. 1981. Interindividual variation and drug interactions with hormonal steroid contraceptives. *Drugs* 1:46–61.
3. Gupta, K., and Ali, M. 1980. Failure of oral contraceptive with rifampicin. *Med. J. Zambia* 15:23.
4. Back, D.J., et al. 1978. The effect of antibiotics on the enterohepatic circulation of ethinylestradiol and norethisterone in the rat. *J. Steroid Biochem.* 9:527–537.
5. O'Brien, T. 1974. Excretion of drugs in human milk. *Am. J. Hosp. Pharm.* 31:847–854.
6. Charles, D. 1981. Antibiotic use during pregnancy. *The Female Patient* 6:67–68.
7. Charles, D. 1980. *Infections in Obstetrics and Gynecology*. Philadelphia: W.B. Saunders Co., pp. 362–425.
8. Beeley, L. 1981. Adverse effects of drugs in later pregnancy. *Clin. Obstet. Gynecol.* 8:275–290.
9. Beeley, L. 1981. Adverse effects of drugs in the first trimester of pregnancy. *Clin. Obstet. Gynecol.* 8:261–273.
10. Beeley, L. 1981. Drugs in breast feeding. *Clin. Obstet. Gynecol.* 8:291–295.
11. Giacoia, G., and Catz, C. 1979. Drugs and pollutants in breast milk. *Clin. Perinatol.* 6:181–196.
12. Platzker, A., Lew, C., and Stewart, D. 1980. Drug administration via breast milk. *Hosp. Pract.* 15:111–122.
13. Bowes, W. 1980. The effect of medications on the lactating mother and her infant. *Clin. Obstet. Gynecol.* 23:1073–1079.
14. Löe, H., and Silness, J. 1963. Periodontal disease in pregnancy. I. Prevalence and severity. *Acta Odontol. Scand.* 21:533–551.

15. Kornman, K.S., and Loesche, W.J. 1980. The subgingival flora during pregnancy. *J. Periodont. Res.* 15:111–122.

16. Jensen, J., Liljemark, W., and Bloomquist, C. 1981. The effect of female sex hormones on subgingival plaque. *J. Periodontol.* 52:599–602.

17. Lindhe, J., and Brånemark, P.I. 1967. Changes in microcirculation after local application of sex hormones. *J. Periodont. Res.* 2:183–193.

18. Lindhe, J., and Brånemark, P.I. 1967. Changes in vascular permeability after local application of sex hormones. *J. Periodont. Res.* 2:259–265.

19. Ojanotko-Harri, A., and Hurttia, M.P. 1987. Progesterone metabolism by rat oral mucosa. III. Participation of granuloma tissue and fibroblasts. *J. Periodont. Res.* 22:37–40.

20. Lundgren, D., Magnussen, B., and Lindhe, J. 1973. Connective tissue alterations in gingivae of rats treated with estrogens and progesterone. *Odontol. Rev.* 24:49–58.

21. Lopatin, D.E., Kornman, K.S., and Loesche, W.J. 1980. Modulation of immunoreactivity to periodontal disease-associated microorganisms during pregnancy. *Infect. Immun.* 28:713–718.

22. Pack, A.R.C., and Thompson, M.E. 1980. Effects of topical and systemic folic acid supplementation on gingivitis in pregnancy. *J. Clin. Periodontol.* 7:402–414.

23. Littner, M.M., et al. 1984. Management of the pregnant patient. *Quintessence Int.* 15:253–257.

24. Steinberg, B.J., and Rose, L.F. 1983. Introduction to the diseases of the endocrine system and the mechanism of action of hormones: Dental Correlations. *Internal Medicine for Dentistry*. St. Louis: The C.V. Mosby Co., pp. 1210–1214.

CHAPTER 20

Legal Considerations

Edwin J. Zinman, D.D.S., J.D.

Fiduciary responsibility

Every dentist is bound by duty to act with fiduciary responsibility (i.e., the responsibility of a guardian) toward his or her patients, so as to minimize the risk of injury and to promote dental health. It is the same duty of reasonable and prudent practice that other fiduciaries owe, such as accountant or lawyer to client, or bank to depositor. In short, a dentist is expected to act as a trustee for the best interest of the patient irrespective of the dentist's own best financial interest. Good documentation and record keeping are an essential part of the responsibility of the dentist.

Customary vs. prudent practice

Prudent practice As a general guideline, prudent practice in dentistry is methods taught in dental schools and continuing education courses and suggested in competent scientific articles, treatises, and textbooks. Prudent guidelines regarding the appropriate standard of treatment care have been promulgated by organizations such as the California Dental Association[1] and the American Academy of Periodontology.[2]

Customary practice Customary practice under a given set of clinical circumstances may constitute evidence of what a reasonable and prudent practitioner would do under the same circumstances.[3] This is never conclusive, however. An arithmetic computation of what the majority of practitioners do in their practices cannot be the only determinant of what a careful and prudent practitioner should do. For instance, some oral surgeons customarily rely exclusively on the panograph for the diagnosis of fractures. Yet it is well known and taught that such tomographic films as the Panorex do not have the diagnostic accuracy of static-beam periapical radiographs.[4-9] Consequently, a radiographically diagnosable fracture could be misdiagnosed as normal. It is for this reason that a practitioner who follows the customary practice of some practitioners, even assuming arguendo a majority, does not necessarily meet the legal standard of care required of a prudent practitioner.

Patients should not dictate the standard of care if it is contrary to the patient's dental and medical interests. For example, if a patient with an existing heart valve arrives at the dentist's office without taking the prescribed dosage of antibiotics 1 hour before the appointment in accordance with the American Heart Association guidelines, the dentist should refuse to treat that patient (see chapter 17). Do not acquiesce if a patient promises to take the prophylactic medication immediately after the appointment and will remember to follow the dentist's directions at the next scheduled maintenance appointment.

A patient cannot legally and validly consent to negligent care. A dentist who permits a patient to override the dentist's best judgment and recommendations violates the standard of care pursuant to the previously described circumstances.

In sum, no matter how many dentists do it wrong, such practices never make it right. A customarily negligent practice does not equate with the standard of care of prudent practitioners.

Proximate cause   By way of defense, a defendant may introduce evidence that, despite the dentist's failure to follow recommended prophylactic administration, SBE (subacute bacterial endocarditis) may have occurred in any event. However, following the recommended regimen reduces the risk of adverse consequences. Therefore, the standard of care should always be followed to reduce the risk, even if such risk is not completely irreducible. While the causal link must be established by expert testimony that the harm was more likely than not a factual result of the dentist's negligence, the issue of causation remains a jury question.[10]

Negligent custom   Examples of customary dental practices that are violations of the **standard of care**, based on the literature, include:

1. Failure to take diagnostic-quality radiographs for caries or periodontal disease[11-13]
2. Improper angulation or development of radiographs[11-13]
3. Diagnosing pathology solely on a wet reading rather than waiting for the image to be finally fixed on the film[11-13]
4. Failure to use a calibrated periodontal probe for the diagnosis of periodontal disease[14-16]
5. Incomplete charting of pathology on dental records[17]
6. Failure to diagnose major oral lesions associated with AIDS (only 22% of dentists routinely used gloves for all patients)[13]
7. Use of experimental drugs, such as Sargenti paraformaldehyde endodontic paste, or N-2[18]
8. Failure to prescribe antibiotics in accordance with recommendations of the American Heart Association[19]
9. Failure to give adequate informed consent[20]
10. Inadequate sterilization techniques[21]

Alternate methods of treatment

Majority vs. minority methods   There can be more than one correct treatment for a given dental infection. It is not negligent to follow a school of thought different from that of the majority of practitioners, provided that the minority method of treatment is adhered to by respected members of the profession.[22] For example, many practitioners do not believe an antibiotic is prophylactically required following tooth extraction if there is no pronounced swelling or fever.[23] Yet some practitioners prescribe prophylactic antibiotic therapy for any residual infection or to prevent secondary infection.[23-25] Where a substantial risk of infection exists, antibiotics are required by all prudent practitioners, irrespective of how many practitioners customarily meet that standard.[23-25] Where a sinus exposure and a risk of oral-antral fistula develops, prudent practice also dictates prophylactic antibiotics.[26]

Foreseeable risk   The legal test is not whether injury has occurred in the past with a given method of treatment, but whether injury is a foreseeable risk or the likelihood of injury is increased by imprudent practice.[27] By analogy, a dog is entitled to one free legal bite before it is determined to have vicious propensities.[28,29] However, dentists are responsible for the "first bite" if such negligent conduct creates a foreseeable, unreasonable risk of harm to the patient.[30]

Duty to refer to a specialist

If immediate blood levels of an antibiotic are required because of life-threatening acute infections, oral antibiotics may be insufficient.[31] Furthermore, studies have shown that approximately one half of all prescriptions are not filled or followed by the patient.[32,33] Consequently, to obtain an adequate blood level of an antibiotic, intramuscular or intravenous antibiotic therapy may be required.[34] If the dentist does not have the antibiotic available in parenteral form, then immediate referral to an oral surgeon or physician for parenteral administration is recommended.

Antibiotics alone may be inadequate therapy for a fulminating space infection with purulence because adequate blood levels of the drug may not effectively reach the site. Accordingly, when fluctuance occurs, surgical incision and drainage procedures, along with bacterial culture/susceptibility tests, should supplement rather than supplant antibiotic therapy (see chapter 4). An untrained generalist should refer such procedures to an oral surgeon; otherwise, the generalist will be held to the standard of care of an oral surgeon, who ordinarily performs incision and drainage.

Duty to obtain medical history

Every patient, whether for emergency treatment or complete examination, can be adequately treated only after an adequate medical history is taken.[35] Examples of such histories have been published in the American Dental Association's *Accepted Dental Therapeutics*.[36] What may have been adequate treatment one year may not be in future

225

years, because the medical history of a patient can change in the interim. **Updating the medical history is therefore required at each recall visit.** Frequently litigated examples are rheumatic fever occurring between dental visits and newly acquired drug allergies.

A *signed* medical history is advisable, but is not legally required. However, in the event that the patient disputes a medical history was taken, a signed and dated history is more credible to a jury than a dentist's memory of past events.

Locality rule

Under former laws and the minority rules of some states, a dentist could be judged only by the standards of other dentists practicing in that locality.[37] This antiquated rule existed because access to current methodology was not equal between rural and urban practitioners. Modern communication and transportation have eliminated the need for the rule. In abolishing the locality rule, the Massachusetts Supreme Court held, "The time has come when the medical profession should no longer be balkanized by the application of varying geographical standards in malpractice cases."[38]

An example of knowledge that is national in scope is the changing standard of care regarding antibiotic prophylaxis in patients with rheumatic valvular defects, intracardiac prosthesis, and prosthetic joint replacements. Thus a dentist who prescribed the 1972 recommended dosage level[39-41] instead of the dosage recommended in 1977[42,43] would be liable for not increasing the frequency or dosage of prophylactic antibiotics, if it could be proven that the onset or severity of subacute bacterial endocarditis was proximately related to the insufficient blood level of the prescribed antibiotic.

Consultation with a physician

A dentist is regarded legally as an expert on pathophysiology of structures of the maxillofacial area. It is therefore important that the dentist be alert to oral implications, such as diminished resistance to infections and resultant poor healing, autoimmune and immunosuppressive diseases, diabetes, and other systemic diseases.

Diabetes   Diabetes can affect the patient adversely during and after surgery by increasing the risk of onset and severity of infection. Consequently, the regulation of a patient's insulin during surgery is a medical decision obtained through consultation with the patient's physician. On the other hand, the decision to prescribe postoperative therapeutic doses of antibiotics is usually determined by the treating dentist, who is more familiar with the nature of the dental surgical procedure than the patient's physician is. Thus, although prophylactic antibiotics are not indicated for routine operative dentistry, dental surgery performed on diabetic or immunocompromised patients carries an increased risk of postoperative infection, usually necessitating prophylactic antibiotic treatment.

Neoplastic and autoimmune diseases   Because disease severity or degree of patient control of a disease can affect the decision for antibiotic coverage for surgical or dental procedures involving the gingiva, physician consultation is suggested for patients suffering from neoplastic or selected autoimmune diseases.

AIDS   Antibiotics for an AIDS patient may interfere with the patient's existing medication and may result in superinfection because of the patient's immunosuppressed status. Accordingly, consultation with the patient's physician with primary treatment responsibilities is required.

Yeast are the main cause of fungal infections in the oral cavity, with *Candida albicans* being the most prevalent species. Dentists should therefore be alert to diagnosing and treating fungal infections with antifungicides in those immunocompromised patients whose yeast flora increases as a result of lowered resistance. In HIV-seropositive patients whose AIDS symptoms have not manifested, the oral cavity can be the first body site affected by *Candida* infections, which represents the premonitor sign of the syndrome.[44]

Failure to consult   A dentist may be negligent in failing to consult with a dental specialist, such as an oral maxillofacial surgeon, or with a physician, when the presenting infection is not controllable initially or postoperatively with oral antibiotics.

For instance, a patient may have been properly prescribed prophylactic oral penicillin for periodontic, endodontic, or impaction surgery. If in 48 hours or more after surgery the patient complains of pain or dysphagia and exhibits submandibular or infraorbital swelling, a consultation with an oral surgeon is mandatory because oral antibiotics would probably be inadequate to control the spreading infection. Proper therapy (oral penicillin) would be modified because of fulminating infection, which could potentially impair the airway, cause blindness, or precipitate a cavernous sinus thrombosis or brain abscess. In such a situation, incision, drainage, and culturing for susceptible microorganisms would be required by the standard of care.

Necessity for culture

In routine treatment   Cultures are not currently used during routine dental treatment. Although once recommended, they are no longer used to verify the sterility of root canal systems—endodontic canals, for example. Proper biomechanical debridement of the root canal is now considered sufficient.[45]

In oral infection   Cultures are still used for cellulitises where initial antibiotic dosage and selection have failed to prevent the infection from invading adjacent tissue spaces, or for the immunocompromised patient whose clinical course cannot be predicted. The spreading infection may be caused by a resistant or arcane microorganism that a culture and susceptibility test, including blood culture, can isolate and identify.

Notwithstanding that penicillin is the drug of choice for oral infections, penicillinase-producing organisms present in an infection may reduce its effectiveness. Culturing can pinpoint the appropriate antimicrobial drug and dosage to be administered under such circumstances.

Although a dentist need not identify the specific etiologic organism before prescribing an antimicrobial drug, he or she is duty-bound to identify the causative organisms if initial antibiotic therapy proves ineffective.[26] Only by identifying the principal pathogenic organisms can selective antibiotic therapy control otherwise resistant microorganisms.

Package inserts

A dentist is legally required to be familiar with current drug package inserts usually replicated in the *Physicians' Desk Reference* or the *Dentists' Desk Reference* for prescribed or dispensed drugs. Standard dental practice also requires such awareness to be updated as new knowledge of deleterious side effects becomes known.

For instance, chloramphenicol was touted originally as the preferred drug for penetrating deep-seated bony infections. Subsequent discovery of aplastic anemias associated with chloramphenicol depreciated its pharmacological value for routine usage. Thus, a dentist who prescribed **chloramphenicol indiscriminately or without just cause** would be legally liable for failure to consider safer alternative antibacterial drugs.

Similarly, prescribing an antibiotic for therapy not approved or recommended in the package insert exposes a dentist to avoidable legal risks.[26,46] Accordingly, if it is known or should be known that the infection is primarily anaerobic, then a drug such as erythromycin would not be as effective as other antimicrobial drugs that specifically are approved and therapeutically preferred for anaerobic organisms.

Dosage

Antibiotics must be prescribed in adequate dosages. Patients should be advised to complete all prescribed antibiotic regimens to militate against the development of resistant strains. Prevalence of increasing resistant strains has resulted in concomitant increases in duration, dosage, and strength of drug prescribed. For instance, 250 mg of penicillin q.i.d. as a therapeutic or prophylactic dose is now outmoded, and a minimum of 500 mg q.i.d., plus the appropriate loading dose of up to 2,000 mg of penicillin should be prescribed. When a dentist fails to prescribe an adequate dosage of antimicrobial, the legal burden of proof that the cause of the infection or its spread was not caused by the lower-than-acceptable prescribed levels may fall upon the dentist.[47]

Informed consent

The legal doctrine of requiring informed consent to inherent and collateral risks of a procedure applies primarily to elective procedures where the therapeutic risks are usually not appreciated by the patient. Specifically, the patient should be told of the benefits and likely risks associated with a drug and the consequences of not taking the prescribed medication. Patient information for several drugs is available from the

American Dental Association and the American Medical Association in the form of tear-out pads for tetracycline, penicillin, and erythromycin.

Reasonable risk   Many states apply an objective standard when informed consent is not given by permitting the jury to consider as a defense whether a reasonable person would have refused antibiotics if informed of the reasonably foreseeable material risks. Therefore, even if the dentist did not advise the patient of the significant risks associated with the antibiotic, if a reasonable person would have taken such risks, then the dentist's nondisclosure to the litigating patient would be exculpated.[48]

Elective vs. nonelective   **Once an infection occurs, the prescribing of antibiotics is principally the doctor's decision rather than a decision of both doctor and patient.** The dentist should stress the risks of spreading infection if the drugs are not taken as prescribed or to completion.

Conversely, prophylactic antibiotic coverage may be considered elective; the risks and benefits are weighed by the patient before prophylaxis proceeds. No discussion of rare or remote risks is generally required, but the predictable short-term risks and serious side effects should be reviewed. If antibiotics are refused the dentist should record the reason on the patient's chart.

Gastrointestinal disturbances are usually self-limiting and short-term. Neuropathies, such as the auditory eighth nerve injury caused by streptomycin, should be considered and discussed before prescribing, since alternative antibiotics with less serious sequellae may offer therapeutically equivalent effectiveness with greater safety.

Oral contraceptives   Antibiotics may theoretically reduce the effectiveness of oral contraceptives. Therefore, although the risk is small, the magnitude of responsibility is great, particularly in the event of a malformed baby requiring lifetime medical care. At least two cases of dental negligence have been settled out of court involving a dentist's failure to warn of the antibiotic inhibition of oral contraceptive effectiveness in pregnancy prevention.[49] *Therefore, in an abundance of caution, a prescribing dentist should provide the warning to women of child-bearing years after first taking the medical history so that this information may be learned and a precautionary warning provided.* Additionally, a dentist may wish to write such warning on the prescription itself so that the pharmacist may include it on the warning label as a double precaution and also as additional evidence that the patient was adequately warned.[49,50]

Case histories

Duty to obtain medical history

Scandalis v. Kaiser[51]   A periodontist was protected from an adverse jury verdict because his records contained a signed medical history in which the patient had denied ever having diabetes. After undergoing one quadrant of periodontal surgery without antibiotics, the patient developed cellulitis and Ludwig's angina. Following hospitalization, the patient died because of the incorrect use of insulin by the hospital staff. Although the case was settled in the middle of trial for $525,000, the periodontist was dismissed from the lawsuit before the trial began since the patient's signed history denying diabetes proved he had acted with due care. In the absence of a signed medical history form, the jury would have had to resolve whether they believed the doctor took a medical history.

Failure to prescribe antibiotics

Butler v. Brady[52]   A 71-year-old male patient went to the office of a dentist who advertised: "Over ninety percent of our work is plates and extractions." The defendant dentist admitted in trial that the advertisement was not true, and that it had been written to attract patients.

The plaintiff was a poorly controlled diabetic who, of his own volition, had discontinued taking insulin 1 month before the extraction. The plaintiff claimed at trial that no inquiry was made of his history of diabetes. Following the extraction of a tooth, the patient developed a massive fulminating infection requiring hospitalization.

The plaintiff contended that he had suffered substantially reduced life expectancy due to kidney damage and would consequently require renal dialysis in the future. The jury verdict was for $400,000, less 20% for the plaintiff's contributory negligence, for a total of $368,000. In lieu of appeal, the plaintiff settled the case for $200,000. However, upon the demise of the plaintiff, which occurred 18 months after the verdict, the widow sued for the wrongful death of her husband. The case is pending.

Willow v. Bingham[53]   Following the extraction of a maxillary first molar, an oral-antral fistula developed. No antibiotics were prescribed for 21 days before an oral surgeon was consulted. The patient underwent a Caldwell-Luc procedure in a failed attempt to close the fistula. Residual chronic sinusitis resulted. The case resulted in a verdict for $70,000.

Snow v. Xavier[54]   A 1981 Massachusetts case involving antibiotic coverage is the largest dental malpractice verdict ever. A general dentist extracted a third molar tooth. When the patient returned with postoperative complications, including signs of infection, no antibiotics were prescribed. The patient subsequently developed spinal meningitis and was comatose for several months. At trial, the plaintiff was 20 years old and suffering the painful and crippling effects of meningitis. The jury awarded $2.75 million. (The largest medical negligence verdict is $29 million for failure to promptly administer antibiotics for bacterial meningitis.[55])

Conclusion

Careful and prudent practice in prescribing antibiotics is the best dental medicine to administer for malpractice prophylaxis. To paraphrase Alexander Pope: To err is human; to err in the use of antibiotics may be harmful but is preventable with due care.

References

1. California Dental Assoc. 1977. *General guidelines for the assessment of clinical quality and professional performance.* (Monograph) Sacramento: CDA.

2. American Academy of Periodontology. 1983. *Guidelines for Periodontal Therapy.* Chicago: AAP.

3. Barton v. Owen, 71 Cal. App. 3d 484, 139 Cal. Rptr. 494 (1977).

4. Report of ADA Council on Dental Materials and Devices. 1977. *J. Am. Dent. Assoc.* 94:147.

5. Christen, A.G., and Segreto, V.A. 1968. Distortion and artifacts encountered in Panorex radiographs. *J. Am. Dent. Assoc.* 77:1096–1101.

6. Mitchel, L.D., Jr. 1963. Panoramic roentgenography. *J. Am. Dent. Assoc.* 66:777–786.

7. Brueggemann, I.A. 1967. Evaluation of the Panorex unit. *Oral Surg. Oral Med. Oral Pathol.* Sept.:348–358.

8. Updegrave, W.J. 1963. Panoramic dental radiography. *Dent. Radiogr. Photogr.* 36(4):76–78.

9. Appelbaum, M. 1983. Differential diagnosis of cervical radiolucencies. *Dent. Radiogr. Photogr.* 56:15.

10. Harlow v. Chin, 405 Mass. 697, 545 N.E. 2d 602 (1989). Harper, F., James, F., and Gray, O. Law of Torts 89-113 (1986).

11. Biedeman, R.W., Johnson, O.N., and Alcox, P.U. 1976. A study to develop a rating system and evaluate dental radiographs submitted to a third party carrier. *J. Am. Dent. Assoc.* 93:1010. (Majority of radiographs not of diagnostic quality.)

12. ADA News. 1975. Accuracy required for proper perio diagnosis. ADA News Nov. 17, p. 8.

13. Abstract of 1990 IADR meeting, reported in *Dental Products*, March 1990.

14. Glavind, C., and Löe, H. 1967. Errors in the clinical assessment of periodontal destruction. *J. Periodont. Res.* 2:180–184.

15. Glazer, S.A. 1972. Reliability of X-ray scores in Navy Periodontal Disease Index. *U.S. Navy Medical* 60:34–37.

16. Morgulis, J. 1979. Developing a periodontal screening evaluation. *Calif. Dent. Assoc. J.* Jan:59.

17. Harney, D. 1973. *Medical Malpractice.* Indianapolis: The Allen Smith Co., p. 286.

18. Zinman, E.J. 1980. Usual and customary versus prudent practice. *J. Tenn. Dent. Assoc.* 60:9.

19. Sadowsky, P., and Kunzil, C. 1989. Usual and customary practice versus the recommendations of experts: Clinical noncompliance in the prevention of bacterial endocarditis. *J. Am. Dent. Assoc.* 118:75.

20. Zinman, E.J. 1976. Advise before you incise. *J. Western Soc. Periodontol.* 24(3):101–115.

21. Silverman, S. 1978. Cold sterilization methods examined. *Dent. Surv.* Oct.:8–10.

22. Barton v. Owen, 71 Cal. App. 3d 484, 139 Cal. Rptr. 494 (1977), Restatement of the Law of Torts, 2d, § 299A (E). (See also: Kruger, G. 1979. *Textbook of Oral Surgery.* 5th ed. St. Louis: The C.V. Mosby Co., p. 173.)

23. Archer, H. 1975. *Oral and Maxillofacial Surgery.* 5th ed. Philadelphia: W.B. Saunders Co., pp. 414, 416.

24. Kruger, G. 1968. *Textbook of Oral Surgery.* 3rd ed. St. Louis: The C.V. Mosby Co., p. 187.

25. Morse, D.R., Furst, M.L., Belott, R.M., Lefkowitz, R.D., et al. 1988. Prophylactic penicillin versus penicillin taken at the first sign of swelling in cases of asymptomatic pulpal-periapical lesions: A comparative analysis. *Oral Surg. Oral Med. Oral Pathol.* 65:228–232.

26. Kruger, G. 1979. *Textbook of Oral Surgery.* 5th ed. St. Louis: The C.V. Mosby Co., p. 284. (See also: Principles of antibiotic therapy v. Indications for antibiotic usage. 1982. *Dent. Drug Serv. Newsl.* 3(4):1.)

27. Crane v. Smith, 23 Cal. 2d 288, 144 P. 2d 356 (1944); 4 Witkin § 496 (1974) Summary of California Law (8th ed.), Torts, p. 496; Restatement, 2d, Torts pp. 289, 291–293; Prosser on Torts (4th ed.) pp. 145–149 (1971).

28. Uccello v. Laudenslayer, 118 Cal. Rptr. 741, 44 Cal. App. 3d 504 (1975).

29. Simpson v. Griggs, 58 Hun. 393, 12 N.Y.S. 162 (1980).

30. Donathan v. McConnell, 193 P. 2d 819, 121 Mont. 230 (1945).

31. Gilman et al. 1980. *Goodman and Gilman's The Pharmacological Basis of Therapeutics.* 6th ed. New York: Macmillan Publishing Co., p. 5.

32. Boyd, J.R., et al. 1974. Drug defaulting. Part 1: Determinants of compliance. *Am. J. Hosp. Pharm.* 31:362.

33. Steward, R.B., and Cluff, L.E. 1973. A review of medication errors and compliance in ambulant patients. *Clin. Pharmacol. Ther.* 13:463.

34. Principles of antibiotic therapy. 1982. Oral versus parenteral routes. *Dent. Drug Serv. Newsl.* 3(6):1–3.

35. Wood, L. 1967. *A Handbook of Dental Malpractice.* Springfield, Ill.: Charles C Thomas, Publishers, p. 33.

36. American Dental Assoc. 1980. *Accepted Dental Therapeutics.* 38th ed. Chicago: ADA, p. 6.

37. Sanderson v. Moline, 499 P. 2d 1281, 7 Wash. App. 439 (1972).

38. Brune v. Belinkoff, 235 N.E. 2d 793 (Mass. 1968).

39. American Heart Assoc. 1977. Prevention of bacterial endocarditis. *Circulation* 56:139A.

40. American Dental Assoc. 1980. Updated labeling for prevention of bacterial endocarditis. *J. Am. Dent. Assoc.* 101:579.

41. Owen, R. 1983. Erythromycin problems. *J. Am. Dent. Assoc.* 106:590.

42. Beeson, P., et al. (eds.) 1979. *Textbook of Medicine.* 15th ed. Philadelphia: W.B. Saunders Co., p. 396.

43. U.S. Food and Drug Administration. 1980. Updated antibiotic labeling for prevention of bacterial endocarditis. *FDA Drug Bull.* 10(2):12.

44. Stenderup, A. 1990. Oral mycology. *Acta Odont. Scand.* 48:3.

45. Cohen, S., and Burns, R. 1980. *Pathways of the Pulp.* 2nd ed. St. Louis: The C.V. Mosby Co., p. 713.

46. Rheingold, P. 1981. *Drug Litigation.* 3rd ed. New York: Practicing Law Institute, pp. 113, 115–123, 320, 321.

47. Stone v. Foster, 164 Cal. Rptr. 901, 106 Cal. App. 3d. 334 (1980).

48. Cobbs v. Grant, 8 Cal. 3d 228, 194 Cal. Rptr. 505 (1973).

49. Antibiotics may interfere with oral contraceptives. *JADA News* 21 (March 5):1, 1990.

50. Morse, D. 1988. Serious sequellae and malpractice in endodontics. *Ann. Dent.* 47(1):33.

51. Scandalis v. Kaiser Permanente, et al., Sacramento Superior Court, Calif. (1972).

52. Butler v. Brady, Alameda County Superior Court, Calif. No. 5074824 (1978).

53. Willow v. Bingham, Sonoma County Superior Court, Calif. No. 78541 (1978).

54. Snow v. Xavier, Somerville Journal, Mass. (1981).

55. Marcelin v. St. John's Episcopal Hospital, N.Y. Sup. No. 24450 (1982).

APPENDIXES

Appendix 1

Typical course of infection management

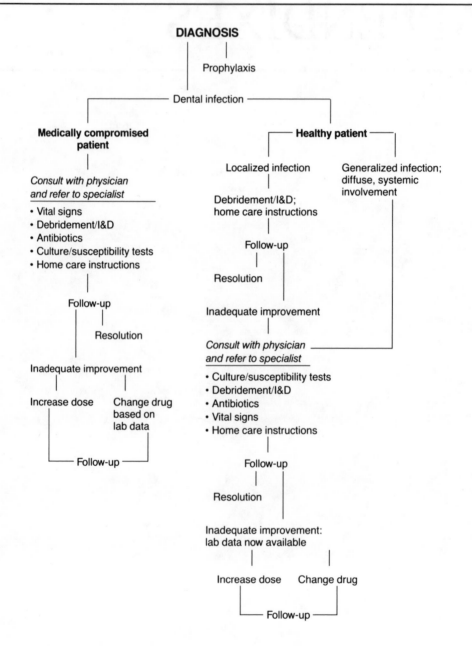

Appendix 2

Local and systemic signs of infection

Local*
- Pain
- Redness
- Edema
- Pus
- Fistula

Systemic†
- Fever
- Elevated vital signs
- Lymphadenopathy
- Malaise
- Elevated leukocyte count

*With most local infections debridement may be sufficient treatment.
†These signs of systemic infection are not universally present. Antibiotic usage is more likely to be necessary when these signs are present.

Appendix 3

Minimum inhibitory concentrations for 90% of anaerobic isolates*

MIC†

Antimicrobial agent	Black-pigmented Bacteroides (40)‡		Fusobacterium (13)		Other gram-negative bacilli (13)§		Veillonella (8)		Gram-positive cocci (11)		Eubacterium (7)	
	Range	90%	Range	90%	Range	90%	Range	90%	Range	90%	Range	90%
Penicillin G	≤0.06–64	0.5	≤0.06–8	0.5	≤0.06–32	4	0.25–0.5	0.5	≤0.06–0.5	0.25	≤0.06–0.5	0.5
Cefadroxil	≤0.06–128	4	0.25–16	8	0.25–64	64	≤0.06–1	0.5	≤0.06–64	16	0.13–64	4
Cephalexin	0.5–32	2	0.5–8	8	0.5–16	16	0.25–1	0.5	0.13–32	8	0.25–64	4
Cephradine	0.25–32	2	0.5–8	8	0.5–32	32	0.13–0.5	0.25	0.5–128	32	0.5–64	16
Cefoperazone	0.13–8	2	≤0.06–8	1	0.25–128	32	0.25–2	2	≤0.06–1	1	≤0.06–2	1
Moxalactam	≤0.06–32	1	0.25–16	16	≤0.06–16	8	≤0.06–2	1	≤0.06–4	2	≤0.06–8	0.5
Sch 29,482	≤0.06–2	0.13	≤0.06–1	1	≤0.06–1	0.5	0.13–0.5	0.25	≤0.06–1	0.5	≤0.06–0.25	0.25
Clindamycin	≤0.06–0.5	0.13	≤0.06–0.25	0.25	≤0.06–2	1	≤0.6–0.25	0.25	≤0.06–0.5	0.5	≤0.06–2	1
Erythromycin	0.13–>128	1	0.5–128	128	≤0.06–2	2	16–64	64	≤0.06–2	2	≤0.06–0.25	0.25
Metronidazole	≤0.06–32	1	≤0.06–0.25	0.25	≤0.06–2	2	0.5–1	1	≤0.06–2	2	≤0.06–64	64
Tetracycline	≤0.06–16	2	≤0.06–16	1	≤0.06–16	1	0.5–2	2	≤0.06–2	1	≤0.06–4	1
Colistin	0.5–>128	>128	0.25–2	1	≤0.06–>128	>128	1–2	1	32–>128	>128	8–>128	>128
Kanamycin	8–>128	>128	0.5–>128	128	0.5–>128	>128	32–>128	64	0.5–>128	128	4–>128	>128
Vancomycin	4–>128	128	16–>128	>128	1–>128	>128	32–>128	>128	0.13–1	1	0.5–2	1

*Source: Sutter et al. (1983).³⁴ Reprinted by permission from the American Society for Microbiology.

†Minimal inhibitory concentrations are expressed in micrograms per milliliter, except penicillin G, which is expressed in units per milliliter. Numbers in parentheses indicate number of strains tested. 90%, MIC inhibiting 90% of isolates.

‡Includes *Bacteroides melaninogenicus, Bacteroides loeschii, Bacteroides denticola, Bacteroides intermedius, Bacteroides corporis, Bacteroides asaccharolyicus, Bacteroides gingivalis,* and the type strain of *Bacteroides macacae.*

§Includes *Bacteroides oralis, Bacteroides ureolyticus,* other *Bacteroides* sp., *Selenomonas* sp., and *Wolinella* sp.

Appendix 4

Minimum inhibitory concentrations for 90% of selected oral isolates*

Microaerophilic and facultative isolates only

MIC†

Antimicrobial agent	Capnocytophaga (17)		Eikenella and Haemophilus (2)‡		Actinomyces (22)§		Arachnia and Propionibacterium (6)§		Lactobacillus (16)§		Streptococcus (39)	
	Range	90%	Range	90%	Range	90%	Range	90%	Range	90%	Range	90%
Penicillin G	0.25–1	1	0.25–0.5	0.5	≤0.6–8	1	≤0.6–0.13	0.13	≤0.06–0.5	0.25	≤0.06–0.5	0.25
Cefadroxil	2–>128	128	8–32	32	≤0.06–2	1	0.13–8	8	≤0.06–1	0.5	0.25–32	16
Cephalexin	1–128	64	4–16	16	≤0.06–2	1	0.25–32	32	≤0.06–2	0.5	0.5–32	16
Cephradine	2–>128	128	8–16	16	0.25–8	4	0.25–64	64	≤0.06–1	1	0.25–32	16
Cefoperazone	0.25–32	8	≤0.06–0.13	0.13	0.13–4	4	0.13–8	8	≤0.06–1	1	≤0.06–4	2
Moxalactam	0.13–16	4	≤0.06	≤0.06	≤0.06–8	4	≤0.06–8	8	0.13–1	0.5	≤0.06–32	8
Sch 29,482	0.25–2	1	0.25–1	1	≤0.06–1	0.5	≤0.06–4	4	≤0.06–0.25	0.25	≤0.06–2	1
Clindamycin	≤0.06–0.13	0.13	16–32	32	≤0.06–4	1	≤0.06–16	16	≤0.06–2	1	≤0.06–128	0.13
Erythromycin	0.13–4	2	1	1	≤0.06–1	0.25	≤0.06–2	2	≤0.06–1	0.5	≤0.06–>128	0.13
Metronidazole	1–32	16	128–>128	>128	0.25–>128	>128	0.5–>128	>128	0.5–>128	>128	128–>128	>128
Tetracycline	0.25–2	2	1	1	0.25–64	4	0.13–2	2	≤0.06–16	1	0.5–128	64
Colistin	128–>128	>128	0.5–1	1	16–>128	>128	128–>128	>128	8–>128	>128	128–>128	>128
Kanamycin	128–>128	>128	1–2	2	8–>128	>128	16–>128	>128	2–128	128	0.5–>128	>128
Vancomycin	0.5–64	32	16–128	128	0.5–8	1	0.25–64	64	0.13–2	1	0.5–2	2

*Source: Sutter et al. (1983).[34] Reprinted by permission from the American Society for Microbiology.

†Concentrations are expressed in micrograms per milliliter, except penicillin G, which is expressed in units per milliliter. Numbers in parentheses indicate number of strains tested. 90%, MIC inhibiting 90% of isolates.

‡One strain each of *Eikenella corrodens* and *Haemophilus aphrophilus*.

§A few strains grew under anaerobic conditions only.

Appendix 5

Peak serum concentrations of antibiotics*

Antimicrobial agent	Route	Serum concentration†
		µg/mL
Penicillins‡	IM/IV	2–200†
Augmentin	Oral	4–7
Benzathine penicillin G	Depot	0.01–0.06
Procaine penicillin G	Depot	0.1–18
Cephalosporins		
Cephalexin	Oral	5–35
Cephadroxyl	Oral	16–28
Cephradine	Oral	5–35
	IV	17–49
Aminoglycosides		
Gentamicin	IV	1–12
Kanamycin	IM	10–25
Streptomycin	IM	10–25
Tetracyclines		
Tetracycline	Oral	1–5
	IV	5–30
Doxycycline	Oral	1–6
Minocycline	Oral	0.7–4.5
Clindamycin	Oral	5–26
Chloramphenicol	Oral	3–12
	IV	20–40
Erythromycin	Oral	<1–10
	IV	5–30
Lincomycin	IV/IM	2–20
Metronidazole	Oral	4–10
Vancomycin	IV	20–50

*Source: Sabath (1980).[35]
†Wide ranges represent the effects of different doses, routes of administration, and preparations. Serum concentrations for oral routes will tend toward the low end of the range given.
‡Penicillins include benzylpenicillin, phenoxymethyl penicillin, amoxicillin, carbenicillin, and cloxacillin.

Appendix 6

Periodontal conditions when microbial samples and analysis should be recommended

I. Adult periodontitis	After conventional periodontal therapy, in unresponsive sites
II. Prepubertal periodontitis	At baseline to check for predominant species and to aid in selection of antimicrobial therapy At different phases of therapy using elimination of predominant species as goal of therapy
III. Juvenile periodontitis	Check for *Actinobacillus actinomycetemcomitans* at the beginning of therapy; use *A. actinomycetemcomitans* elimination as goal of therapy
IV. Rapidly progressing periodontitis	After conventional periodontal therapy, in unresponsive sites to aid in selection of antimicrobial therapy; use elimination of predominant pathogens as goal of therapy
V. Periodontitis associated with systemic diseases	Use elimination of predominant pathogens as goal of therapy
VI. Necrotizing ulcerative periodontitis	After conventional periodontal therapy, in unresponsive sites
VII. Refractory periodontitis	After conventional therapy to aid in selection of antimicrobial therapy; use elimination of predominant pathogens as goal of therapy

Appendix 7

Common errors in antibiotic therapy

1. Viral infections cannot be treated with antibiotics.
2. Ineffective levels of the appropriate drug are administered.
3. A drug that has no established specific effectiveness is prescribed.
4. The infecting agent is not documented.
5. Toxic agents are used when less toxic medication would suffice.
6. Expensive drugs are prescribed when effective inexpensive drugs would suffice.
7. Antibiotic therapy is changed too rapidly and incorrectly, assuming therapeutic failure prior to correcting all contributing factors.
8. Cultures are not taken and susceptibility tests are not obtained.
9. The patient's progress is not monitored.

Appendix 8

Why antibiotic therapy may fail

1. The patient does not comply with the prescription.
2. The dose prescribed is insufficient, or it is prescribed or taken for an insufficient duration.
3. An inappropriate antibiotic is prescribed.
4. The antibiotic is taken simultaneously with an interfering drug, e.g., an antacid with a tetracycline.
5. Drainage is inadequate or necrotic tissues have not been located and removed.
6. The predominant causative bacteria are resistant, resistant strains emerge, or the tissues become secondarily infected with resistant bacteria.
7. The antibiotic fails to reach the infected site (osteomyelitis).
8. A duct, such as a salivary gland, is obstructed or there is an open portal, such as for a urinary catheter or intravenous line.
9. Poor host response, such as malabsorption, is encountered due to a systemic disease.
10. The patient is reacting to a foreign body, such as a transplanted organ or an implant.

Appendix 9

Average oral doses recommended for adults

Assumes 150-pound patient with normal renal and hepatic functions. Actual doses vary with severity of infection.

Antibiotic	Usual dose
Penicillins	
Ampicillin	250–500 mg q6h
Amoxicillin	250–500 mg q6h
Augmentin	250–500 mg q6h
Bacampicillin	400–800 mg q12h
Penicillin G	400,000–600,000 units q6h
Penicillin V	500 mg q6h
Oxacillin	500 mg q6h
Nafcillin	250 mg–1 gr q4–6h
Cloxacillin	500 mg q6h
Dicloxacillin	500 mg q6h
Cephalosporins	
Cephalexin	250–500 mg q6h
Cefaclor	250 mg q6h
Cephadrine	500 mg q6h
Tetracyclines	
Tetracycline HCl	250 mg q6h
Doxycycline	200 mg initially, then 100 mg q12h
Minocycline	200 mg initially, then 100 mg q12h
Erythromycins	
Erythromycin base	250–500 mg q6h
Erythromycin ethylsuccinate	400 mg q6h
Clindamycin	300 mg initially, then 150 mg q8h
Metronidazole	250 mg q8h

Appendix 10

Average doses recommended for children
Actual doses are based on infection severity, child's age, and renal and hepatic clearances.

Antibiotic	Usual dose*		
Ampicillin	50 mg/kg/d (For severe infections the drug should be administered parenterally.)		
Cephalexin	25–50 mg/kg in divided doses (In severe infections the dose can be doubled.)		
Clindamycin, oral†	15–25 mg/kg/d in 3–4 doses; more severe infections, 25–40 mg/kg/d in 3–4 doses, with medical consultation		
Erythromycin (base)‡	30–50 mg/kg/d in divided doses (Doses can be doubled in more severe infections.)		
Erythromycin ethylsuccinate‡	Body weight		Daily dose
	Less than 10 lb		30–50 mg/kg/d 15–25 mg/lb/d
	10–15 lb		200 mg
	16–25 lb		400 mg
	25–50 lb		800 mg
	51–100 lb		1,200 mg
	More than 100 lb		1,600 mg
Penicillin G, oral; and Penicillin V	15–50 mg (25,000–90,000 units)/kg/d in 3–6 divided doses		
Tetracycline HCl	More than 8 years of age: 25–50 mg/kg or 10–20 mg/lb, divided into 4 doses		

*kg refers to child's weight.
†Taken with a full glass of water.
‡Taken before meals.

Appendix 11

Patient-applied local delivery of antibacterial therapy

Advantages	Disadvantages
• No gastric upset	• Difficulty retaining therapeutic levels at site—agent is easily dissolved, diluted, or washed away by saliva
• No alteration of the protective normal flora present at sites distant from the affected area	• Risk of allergy or sensitivity in host reactions
• Should not encourage the transfer of multiple antibiotic resistance between intestinal bacteria	• Produces pulses and large fluctuations in concentration
• Allows concentrated delivery of agents to the affected site without dilution throughout the entire body	• Requires frequent administration
• May be self-administered by the patient	• Requires patient compliance

Appendix 12

Common types of controlled-release delivery devices

- Reservoirs *without* rate-controlling system
  Example: hollow fibers filled with agent. Release of agent is determined simply by diffusion out of the reservoir.

- Reservoirs *with* rate-controlling system
  Example: microcapsules filled with agent. Rate is controlled by solid or microporous polymer membrane. A single dosage might contain different microcapsules with varying release rates.

- Monolithic systems
  Example: agent is dispersed in inert polymeric matrix. Active ingredient is released dependent on the concentration gradient.

- Laminated systems
  Example: multiple layers of polymers with different diffusion characteristics. Central layers may be the agent reservoir with surrounding layers that limit the diffusion rate.

Appendix 13

Common drug interactions*

Drug	Drug	Interaction
Cephalosporins	Gentamicin	Additive, nephrotoxic
	Lasix	Possible increase in nephrotoxicity
	Probenecid	May reduce renal clearance of cephalosporins
Erythromycin	Theophylline	Increases theophylline levels with potential toxicity
Erythromycin	Penicillin(s)	May decrease effectiveness of penicillin(s)
Neomycin	Digoxin	Decreases gastrointestinal absorption of digoxin
	Penicillin V	Oral neomycin decreases absorption of penicillin V
Clindamycin	Erythromycin	Compete for the same protein binding sites
Metronidazole	Alcohol, ethyl	Decreases desire to drink; "Antabuse" reaction to alcohol
	Disulfiram	Psychotic episodes and confusional states may occur
Penicillins	Tetracyclines	May interfere with the bacteriocidal effect of penicillin
	Probenecid Butazolidin	May potentiate penicillin's effects
	Coumadin	May potentiate coumadin's effect
	Tandearil	May potentiate tandearil's effects
	Aspirin	May potentiate penicillin's effects
Tetracycline	Coumadin	Increases anticoagulation
	Feosol Maalox Mylanta Milk products NaHCO$_3$	Decreases effectiveness through absorption and inhibition
	Penicillin(s)	May decrease effectiveness of penicillin

*There is a possibility of superinfection with steroid administration and antibiotics. Bacterostatic antibiotics can decrease the effectiveness of bacterocidal antibiotics.

Appendix 14

Potency of commonly used topical antimicrobial agents*

Agent	Commercial form	Available concentration (μg/mL)	Gram-positive MIC 90 μg/mL†	Gram-negative MIC 90 μg/mL‡	Potency§	Reference
Cetylpyridinium chloride	Scope, Cepacol (Dow Chemical Co)	50	10,000	N/A	Low	1
Chlorhexidine	Peridex (Procter & Gamble)	1,200	32	4	Hi	2
Sanguinarine	Viadent	150	8	4	Hi	3
Sodium fluoride (daily rinse)	Fluorigard	500	2,048	256	Low	4
Thymol	Listerine	600	15,000	N/A	Low	5

*Adapted from Goodson (1989).[6]
†The concentration of drug required to inhibit growth of 90% of the gram-positive organisms tested.
‡The concentration of drug required to inhibit growth of 90% of the gram-negative organisms tested.
§Potency: Hi = MIC^{90} well below applied concentration.
      Moderate = MIC^{90} close to applied concentration.
      Low = MIC^{90} well above applied concentration.

Appendix 15

Common uses of chlorhexidine rinses

Adjunctive supragingival plaque control

- In the management of recurrent or persistent gingivitis
- Following oral surgery/periodontal surgery
- Following crown preparation and during period that provisional restorations are worn
- For physically or mentally handicapped patients

Treatment and control of oral mucosal infections

- Rampant caries
- Gingivitis in immunocompromised patients (e.g., HIV gingivitis) (see chapter 18)
- Prevention and control of mild candidiasis in immunocompromised patients (see chapter 18)
- Aphthous ulcers

Adjunctive control of bacterial recolonization

- In association with treatment of periodontitis
- In association with systemic controlled-release antibiotic treatment of subgingival bacteria

Appendix 16

Antifungal agents for treatment for oral candidiasis

Agent	Available form	Recommended use
Nystatin	Topical: Mycostatin pastilles	Dissolve one pastille 5 times daily for 14 d
	Nystatin Oral Suspension	Swish with 4–6 mL (400,000–600,000 units) 4 times daily for 14 d. Retain in mouth for 2 min before swallowing. Continue treatment for at least 48 h after symptoms have disappeared.
Clotrimazole	Topical: Mycelex troches	Dissolve 1 troche 5 times daily for 14 d
Ketoconazole	Systemic: Nizoral	One tablet (200 mg) daily for 14 d
Fluconazole	Systemic: Diflucan	Two (100-mg) tablets the first day then one tablet daily for a minimum total treatment of 14 d

Appendix 17

Chronic acyclovir therapy to suppress recurrent herpetic episodes

Acyclovir (Zovirax) 200-mg tablets:

- Take 1 tablet 5 times daily for the first 3 d, then
- Take 1 tablet 2 to 4 times daily for 6 mo
- Reevaluate after 6 mo and discontinue therapy
- Chronic suppressive therapy may be reinstituted if patient is stable and has decreased incidence of herpetic episodes after stopping therapy but then the episodes reactivate months or years later

Appendix 18

Emergency treatment of allergic reaction

Immediate allergic reaction

1. Maintain airway, give O_2 6 L/min by mask
2. Call for medical assistance
3. Administer 0.2–0.3 cc of 1:1,000 epinephrine subcutaneously
4. If indicated (condition worsens) administer 50 mg Benadryl IM or IV
5. If indicated (condition worsens) administer 125 mg Sol-u-Medrol IM or IV
6. If condition continues to deteriorate, repeat epinephrine administration 10 min after initial dose

Delayed reaction

Oral antihistamines may be sufficient treatment

Appendix 19

Primary systemic antibiotics for adjunctive treatment of endodontic infections

Penicillin VK
    Drug of first choice
    Confirm no allergies to penicillin

Dosage:
Load with 1,000 mg
Then 500 mg every 6 h for 7–10 d

Doxycycline or minocycline
    Drug of second choice
    Gastrointestinal upset is common

Dosage:
Load with 200 mg
Then 100 mg every 6 h for 7 d

Erythromycin
    Drug of choice with patients allergic to
    penicillin
    Gastrointestinal upset
    Not effective against some oral anaerobes
    Use enteric coated form

Dosage:
Load with 1,000 mg
Then 500 mg every 6 h for 7 d

Appendix 20

Antibiotic selection summary for odontogenic infections

Drug of choice: Penicillin V

If patient is penicillin allergic:

- Erythromycin—bacteriostatic
- Cephalosporin—bactericidal; *note:* may produce allergic reactions in 5%–15% of the patients allergic to penicillin
- Tetracyclines—bacteriostatic; use if allergic to penicillins and cephalosporins and cannot tolerate erythromycin

Chronic infection, inadequate response to penicillin:

- Clindamycin
- Metronidazole
- Metronidazole + penicillin in more severe infections

Appendix 21

Principles of managing odontogenic infections

Step 1: Determine severity

- History of onset and progression
- Physical examination of area
  (1) character and size of swelling
  (2) presence of trismus

Step 2: Evaluate host defenses

- Diseases that compromise the host
- Medications that compromise the host

Step 3: Surgical treatment

- Remove the cause of infection
- Drain pus
- Relieve pressure

Step 4: Antibiotic choice

- Determine:
  (1) most likely causative organisms based on history
  (2) host defense status
  (3) allergy history
  (4) previous drug history
- Prescribe drug properly

Step 5: Followup

- Confirm treatment response
- Evaluate for side effects and secondary infections

Appendix 22

Chemotherapeutic agents in restorative dentistry

Purpose	Agent	Regimen	Instructions
Gingival enhancement in fixed prosthodontics	0.12% chlorhexidine gluconate (Peridex)	15 mL bid 30 s rinse; start 2 weeks before tooth preparation, continue for 2 weeks after final cementation	Brush and floss teeth first. Rinse with chlorhexidine 15 mL bid for 30 s and expectorate; do not rinse, eat, or drink for 30 min
Long-term maintenance of extensive fixed prosthodontics	0.4% stannous fluoride gel/over-the-counter sodium fluoride rinses	Fluoride gel placed in stent/daily rinsing	Once a day place gel in stents, hold both maxillary and mandibular stents in mouth for 4 min; expectorate excess gel; do not rinse, eat, or drink for 30 min
Long-term maintenance of periodontal-prostheses	0.12% chlorhexidine gluconate (Peridex)	Apply with interproximal brush or dilute 3:1 for irrigation device once daily	Apply with interproximal brush or irrigation device
Denture stomatitis (candidiasis)	Nystatin pastilles	400,000–600,000 units qid, continue for 48 h after symptoms have resolved	Suck on pastilles until completely dissolved qid. Continue for 48 h after symptoms have resolved
Denture stomatitis (candidiasis)	Ketoconazole	200–400 mg/d	200–400 mg/d
Severe denture stomatitis (candidiasis)	Consult with patient's physician on therapeutic options		
Recurrent herpes labialis	Topical acyclovir (Zovirax, 5% ointment)	Apply as needed to affected areas	Apply 5% ointment as needed to affected areas
Systemic herpes infection (herpes simplex virus)	Acyclovir (Zovirax)	IV 250 mg/m^2 q8h for 7 d	IV 250 mg/m^2 q8h for 7 d
		Oral 200–400 mg 5 times/d for 7–10 d	Oral 200–400 mg 5 times/d for 7–10 d

Appendix 23

Treatment of postoperative implant complications

After implant placement

Wound infection
- Drainage
- Antibiotic susceptibility testing
- Penicillin* 500 mg q6h for ≥ 7 d
- If no improvement within 2 d:
  —change antibiotic according to susceptibility test results
  or
  —remove implant
- In fulminant cases:
  —admit to hospital for IV antibiotic therapy

Flap dehiscence
- Eliminate cause
- Excise tissue around dehiscence
- If implant is exposed:
  —0.12% chlorhexidine 15 mL q12h

No primary osseointegration
- Remove implant

After uncovering implants (two-stage systems only)

Wound infection
- Mechanical debridement and
- 0.12% chlorhexidine rinse
- If fluctuance:
  —drainage
  —antibiotic susceptibility testing
  —penicillin* 500 mg q6h for ≥ 7 d
- If no improvement within 2 d:
  —change antibiotic according to susceptibility test results
- If implant is mobile, remove it
- In fulminant cases:
  —admit to hospital for IV antibiotic therapy

*Amoxicillin or Augmentin may also be administered, depending on individual circumstances and clinical judgment.

Appendix 24

Patients at-risk from bacteremia-induced infections*

Very-high-risk, high-risk, and intermediate-risk patients should receive antibiotic prophylaxis. No chemoprophylaxis is normally required for low-risk patients.† Other indications may include orthopedic prosthetic appliances, hemodialysis, and impaired host defenses.

Antibiotic prophylaxis indicated

Very high risk

Previous episode of infective endocarditis
Heart valve prosthesis
Coarctation of the aorta
Indwelling catheter left side of heart

High risk

Rheumatic heart disease
Other acquired valvular heart disease
Congenital heart disease
   Ventricular septal defect
   Patent ductus arteriosus
   Tetralogy of Failot
   Complex cyanotic heart disease
   Systemic-pulmonary artery shunt
   Indwelling catheter right side of heart
   Mitral valve surgery
   Mitral valve prolapse with murmur
   Ventriculoatrial shunts for hydrocephalus
   Idiopathic hypertrophic subaortic stenosis

Intermediate risk

Tricuspid valve disease
Assymetric septal hypertrophy

Other at-risk patients

Orthopedic prosthetic devices
Immunosuppression
Hemodialysis

Antibiotic prophylaxis usually not indicated†

Low risk

Mitral valve prolapse without murmur
Coronary artery disease
Atherosclerotic plaque
Previous myocardial infarction

Coronary bypass

Indwelling cardiac pacemakers
Congenital pulmonary stenosis
Uncomplicated secundum septal atrial defect
Six months or longer after surgery for:
   Ligated ductus arteriosus
   Autogenous vascular grafts
   Surgically closed atrial or septal defects
     (without Dacron patches)

*Reprinted with permission of Pallasch.[10]
†Check with patient's physician.

Appendix 25

Recommended antibiotic regimens for prevention of infective endocarditis during dental and upper respiratory procedures

---

Adult dosage

Standard regimen

2 g of penicillin V 1 h preoperatively; 1 g, 6 h after the initial dose.

Penicillin-allergic

1.6 g of erythromycin ethylsuccinate 1.5 h preoperatively; 0.8 g, 6 h after the initial dose.

(If base or sterate forms of erythromycin are used, adequate blood levels will probably not be reached in the initial 1 h preoperative recommendation.) 1 g erythromycin 1 h preoperatively; 500 mg 6 h after the initial dose.

Special regimen

Ampicillin 1–2 g IM or IV plus gentamicin 1.5 mg/kg IM or IV 30–60 min preoperatively. 1 g of penicillin V 6 h after the initial dose or repeat the parenteral regimen 8 h later.

Penicillin-allergic

Vancomycin 1 g IV administered slowly over 1 h starting 1 h before treatment; no postoperative dose required.

Children's dosage

Standard regimen

>60 lb—adult dosage
<60 lb—one half the adult dose
1 h before the procedure and
6 h after the initial dose

Penicillin-allergic

20 mg/kg of erythromycin ethylsuccinate 1.5 h before the procedure and 6 h after the initial dose

Special regimen

Ampicillin 50 mg/kg IM or IV 30–60 min before procedure then repeat once 8 h later. Gentamicin 20 mg/kg IM or IV 30–60 min before procedure then repeat once 8 h later either parenterally or orally (1 g of penicillin V).

Penicillin-allergic

Vancomycin 20 mg/kg IV infused over 1 h, beginning 1 h before procedure.

Appendix 26

Relative risks of infective endocarditis based on underlying cardiac lesions and American Heart Association recommended protocol

At-risk level	Recommended protocol
Patients at high risk:	Special regimen (see **Table 17.3**)
• Previous history of IE • Prosthetic heart valve • Intravascular prostheses • Coarctation of the aorta	
Patients at significant risk:	Standard regimen (see **Table 17.3**)
• Rheumatic valvular diseases • Acquired valvular disease • Congenital heart disease	
Patients at minimal risk:	Standard regimen (see **Table 17.3**)
• Transvenous pacemaker • History of rheumatic fever without rheumatic heart disease	
Patients with minimal risk who do not usually require prophylaxis:*	Standard regimen (see **Table 17.3**)
• Incurred or functional murmur • Uncomplicated atical septal defects • Coronary artery bypass graft operations	

*Check with patient's physician.

Appendix 27

Antimicrobial therapy with HIV infection and organ transplantation

Infection/virus	Treatment
Odontogenic	Penicillin VK 2 g orally 1 h before treatment and then 1 g 6 h later (treat for longer duration if active infection or major surgical procedure involved)
HIV gingivitis/ periodontitis	Vigorous scaling and root planing and 0.12% chlorhexidine rinse 7 mL for 30 s 3 times/d for 7 d
	If above is unsuccessful, metronidazole 250-mg tablets 4 times/d for 7 d
Candidiasis	*Nystatin suspension:* swish in mouth for 2 min and swallow 4 times/d for 14 d
	Clotrimazole troches: dissolve 1 troche in mouth 5 times/d for 14 d
	Ketoconazole: take 1 tablet daily for 14 d
Herpes simplex	*Acyclovir IV:* 5 mg/kg given over 1 h 3 times/d for 5–7 d
	Acyclovir capsules: take 1 capsule 5 times/d for 7–20 d
	Acyclovir prophylaxis for organ transplantation: acyclovir capsules 3 times/d beginning the day of transplant and continue for 30 d

Index

255

Index

Index